Chapter 1: The Prostate and How it Works

Are you aware of the 10 incredible functions of the prostate? It is no wonder that it is vital for men's health as well as the reproduction of the species.

The Prostate's Purpose

Gland

The primary function of the prostate is to produce some alkaline seminal fluids and secrete them during ejaculation (30 to 35% of the ejaculate). The prostate fluid is milky white in color and alkaline. It helps the sperm survive the acidic vaginal environment. Since glands secrete something, the prostate is considered a gland.

Mix Master

To transport the sperm from the testicles, the prostate mixes its fluids and those of the seminal vessels. These fluids flow through the prostate and into the urethra during the ejaculation. The urethra acts as both the semen tube and the urine tube from bladder during ejaculation. Both fluids exit the penis at different times. The prostatic urethra is the section of the urethra running through the prostate gland. It measures approximately 3cm (1 1/2 inches) in length.

The prostate-specific antigen (PSA), a fluid that is produced in the prostate, plays a crucial role in allowing the sperm into the uterus. It keeps the semen in liquid state. It works by preventing the seminal fluid's clotting enzyme from gluing the semen to the woman's cervix. This is located next to the uterus entry inside the vagina. PSA disintegrates this glue with its own enzyme, so the sperm can enter the uterus to immunize an egg.

This is the same PSA that's tested during the PSA Blood Test. It's a controversial test due to the numerous factors that can affect the results.

Muscle

The prostate is also a muscle which pumps the semen through the penis, allowing it to enter the vagina and aid the sperm in reaching the cervical area.

AH!

The pumping action of your prostate is a bonus for males. It makes sex more attractive and helps procreation.

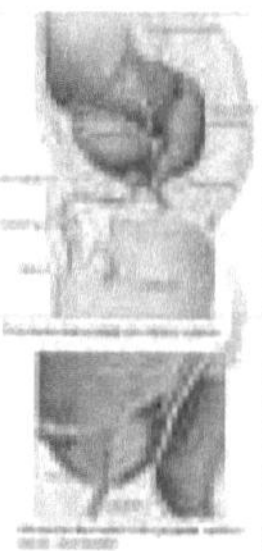

G-spot

The male G-spot is located in the prostate.
If a man is open to the idea of prostate stimulation, he may experience a strong sexual response and an intense orgasm. Longer orgasms, and even "injaculations," where no semen are expelled, can be possible by controlling ejaculation at your prostate. To contain sexual energy, advanced Tantric and Taoist sexual practices use this method.

Filter

Also, the prostate filters and removes toxic substances to protect the sperm. This increases the chances of immunization and ensures that men are able to conceive with the best quality sperm. This is the most important function of the prostate and can also be one reason there is an increasing number of cases of prostate cancer and other diseases.

Erections

Erections can be caused by the prostate erection nervous system. These nerves cause the penis to swell with blood flow, resulting in an erection.

According to the Macmillan Cancer Support charity in the UK, men with prostate cancer are more likely than those without it to experience impotence or erectile dysfunction. Side effects can result from many medical procedures, such as radiation and hormone treatments. Erectile problems can be caused by permanent damage to these nerves, which attach to the sides and prostate.

According to The Belfast Telegraph, 160,000 men in the UK who are being treated with prostate cancer are also experiencing erectile dysfunction. They had greater difficulty getting and maintaining erections after they received medical treatment.

Officials at Macmillan Cancer Support stated that almost two-thirds (33%) of prostate cancer patients report inability to erection due to their treatment.

Professor Jane Maher is the chief medical officer for the UK's cancer charity. She stated, "The sheer number of men affected shows that there is a need to have careful discussions before treating them."

Secretions

The protective role of the prostate gland from infections in the urinary tract is also a very important one.

Valves

The bladder is surrounded by the prostate (the prostatic tube). It controls the flow of urine. Except for when urine is released by urination, it prevents urine leaving the bladder. It prevents urine from damaging the ejaculate in orgasm.

This is done with two small muscles, called sphincters. They are gatekeepers that control and regulate the dual-purpose Urethra tube. These gatekeepers make sure the correct fluids flow at the right times --urination and ejaculation. Not a bad design!

The bladder and upper parts of the prostate intersect at the sphincter. This is the internal upper sphincter. It prevents urination from occurring until it is time to go. Additionally, seminal fluid does not shoot backwards into bladders during ejaculation if it functions properly.

Semen is forced back into the bladder when this sphincter becomes damaged.

It eventually stops with normal urination. Retrograde ejaculation is another side effect of prostate surgery. There is no chance of seeding a female then!

The external lower sphincter, located at the base the prostate, is also subject to our control. It prevents us from dribbling after we pee and allows us to delay urinating when it is not convenient. Incontinence occurs when the control of one sphincter is lost and urine flows or leaks uncontrollably. This causes many men with prostate problems to have to use adult diapers.

If you have enough Kegel muscle control and the ability to shut off the flow, it's possible to control the lower sphincter. Either of these sphincter muscles can block urine until you feel the need to pee. When the time is right, let it flow.

BPH, or an enlarged prostate, can cause urination difficulties and other unpleasant symptoms. Side effects of BPH surgery that removes part of the prostate may include incontinence and retrograde ejaculation.

Hormones

The 5-alpha-reductase enzyme is a key enzyme in the prostate gland. This enzyme converts testosterone into DHT.

(dihydrotestosterone), which is at least ten times more powerful than simple testosterone. The powerful hormone DHT serves many purposes, including male sexual drive. As men age, the amount of DHT produced can be affected by a buildup of prostate toxins.

DHT and testosterone were mistakenly viewed as the culprit hormones for prostate problems. They are often linked to an excessive rise in male estrogen levels. This can lead to medical interventions that have serious side effects, including a lack of libido.

The high levels of estrogens found in food and milk products, including factory and commercial meats, dairy products and body-care products, causes them to rise. It can even be found in municipal water, and certain plastic food packaging.

Prostate disease is a serious condition that can cause havoc to a man's overall health. It would be a good idea for men to take steps to improve their prostate health. A poor prostate health can have a huge impact on sexual function as well as daily urination.

The prostate is a powerful gland that has huge implications on men's lives!

It is a great design! This is in direct contradiction to the jokes that many urologists make about where the prostate should go.

Take a look at all its incredible functions. Its perfect design is what makes the prostate so amazing. There are on-off switches that control the flow of penis fluids, such as urine or ejaculate. We would have two separate organs otherwise. These complications are for sex, and one for urination. You could probably have two penises but they would be incompatible at the wrong time!

We have a wonderful system. Problems arise when we get the wrong inputs, and then we start to experience prostate problems! All the prostate is doing is performing one of its key functions--eliminating toxins from the ejaculate to protect the sperm. We are inundated by toxins, which can lead to health problems.

Keep in mind how close your prostate is to the bladder, rectum and kidneys. Because of their proximity, the prostate can absorb toxins easily from these organs. This is why diets in the broadest sense of the term are so important for the health and well-being of the prostate.

The rectum and urinary tract are the organs that eliminate most of the toxins and waste products in our bodies. Higher levels of toxicity in the body will result in higher levels of toxicity in the urine and feces.
Because the prostate is so close to these organs, it is very vulnerable

to toxicity accumulation. This happens because urine flows through the prostate and toxins are leaked from the bladder.

Prostate Health: Herbs for Treating Inflammation by M. Vertolli, vitalitymagazine.com/article/prostate-health-herbs-for-treatinginflammation/

What is the solution? You can add more toxic substances to your body by taking meds that have severe side effects and pose a risk of cancer. Radiate and chemicalize the prostate, in case it is cancer. If you believe that this is the best way to go, you're lying to yourself.

You will first experience side effects like incontinence (dribbling, diapers and impotence) or impotence ("troubles getting up). You will then experience a recurrence in prostate conditions, as you are adding trauma to your body. Even if your prostate is removed, you can still get prostate cancer. Yes, cancer can spread to the area where it was once located.

I believe that the only way to solve your problem is to either stop the actual causes or to change the situation now in order to prevent any further problems.

Are you too busy to make any changes? Life will eventually force you to make changes. The ultimate wealth is health. What are you left with if your health is poor? You can make a great investment in your health and enjoy it for the rest of you life. A healthy lifestyle is one that encourages vitality, not chronic illness.

Take care of your prostate. All the dimensions of food that we will be discussing should be considered when you eat. You will learn about whole foods and real food that can provide you with many benefits.

Conclusion

After I realized how vitally important the prostate was, I could see how disease can affect our lives and how conventional treatment for prostate problems can negatively impact our lives.

A healthy prostate is essential for a healthy body.

In Chapter 2, you will learn how early diagnosis of prostate cancer can lead to men becoming more likely to develop it.

Chapter 2: Causes of Prostate Cancer

You Are The Cause!

A prostate problem is a sign that your body is suffering from something. There are many causes for disease.

This insight should be the foundation of all medical practice. Unfortunately, it is not. Western medical practice only focuses on the symptom or condition. This is what is called symptomatic medicine. It fails to find the root cause of the condition, allowing healing to occur at the most profound level.

They will often blame their family history or genes for the development of prostate cancer. You won't believe it! Yes, families can have a history. But I believe it is the food we eat and the lack of exposure to the sun that are the key factors in prostate cancer.

Even if you have a genetic disposition to prostate cancer, the impact of your daily food and other inputs on your cellular health is far greater. Your body's cells are completely replaced every 7 years. So your inputs can have a huge impact. That was my 3-year old granddaughter's favorite phrase for a long while!).

While some cancers can be influenced greatly by genetic defects inherited from the parents, epigenetics is proving that your genetic code may not be as predeterministic than previously believed.

The way your genes are expressed is up to you. You have a lot of control over how your genes express and suppress your genetic data. This includes the environment where they are found, the availability or lack of toxins, nutrients and your thoughts and feelings. These factors can affect hormones and other chemicals in the body. This article will explain more.

Genetic Testing for Breast Cancer, Radical Masectomy and Genetic Testing for Breast Cancer--Are You?

Are Women being misled into a false sense of security? by Dr. Mercola, http://articles.mercola.com/sites/articles/archive/2013/05/27/angelin ajolie-double-mastectomy.aspx

Don't worry about your family history or genes--which are out of your control. Instead, change what you can and get started now.

You can often end up with unpleasant side effects if you don't find the cause of prostate cancer. The most common side effects are incontinence and sexual problems. Cancer can also recur later on or in another part of the body. It is not possible to change the conditions that led to the problem.

Traditional Chinese Medicine recognizes that each organ has a complementing organ. If one organ is damaged by disease and not properly treated, it will often lead to the death of another.

Over thousands of years, we evolved based on real food and not artificial or contaminated food that is so prevalent in our modern diets.

Can it be possible to eat healthy foods today that contain chemical ingredients we can't pronounce? Are foods made with artificial fertilizers, pesticides, and herbicides health-enhancing? The answer is yes!

These toxins can build up over time, sometimes for decades, and eventually cause chronic diseases. Chronic disease is the result of the body's last ditch effort to eliminate toxins and protect itself from the onslaught.

Prostate disease has become a major problem in the West. The prostate is located between the bladder and colon, which are the two main organs of elimination. Your urine and feces will be more toxic if you eat a toxic diet. These toxins can easily be absorbed by your prostate.

Your urine actually passes through your prostate as it heads out. Furthermore, your rectum lies adjacent to your prostate and is separated only by the thin rectal wall. A trained urologist can assess the condition of your prostate by performing the famous digital rectal exam.

Men often experience prostate problems at midlife due to the slow progression of prostate disease: enlargements, infections and cancers.

Let's look at the role of sleep in all this. Poor sleeping habits = higher cancer risk. A study published in Cancer, Epidemiology, Biomarkers and Prevention showed that prostate cancer was twice as likely for men who have difficulty sleeping than those who sleep well. Here's an excerpt taken from an article.

The association was stronger in advanced prostate cancer cases, where the risk of developing the disease was greater. . . . Lara Sigurdardottir (Ph.D.), is the lead researcher. She believes that "if our results are confirmed by future studies, sleep could become a potential target of intervention to reduce the risk for prostate cancer."

Chronic sleep problems can lead to insulin resistance and decreased melatonin levels, which in turn can increase your chance of developing cancer. Your insulin resistance is affected by your sleep habits. This means that no matter how healthy you eat or how active you are, your health could be at risk. See Dr. Mercola's article, Research Again Confirms the Links Between Poor Sleep, Weight Gain, Cancer and Other Health Issues.

It is much easier to prevent damage than reverse it. Proper nutrition for the prostate is essential. You don't have to wait too long to reap the rewards. Stop eating toxic foods. Next, you need to eat healthy food.

Because your body is unable to cope with constant exposure from poor quality foods, toxic foods can have an impact on your quality of sleep.

Our health and well-being is determined by our food choices. Your health and the condition of your prostate are directly affected by your diet. Poor diet, lack of sunlight, electromagnetic fields from smart meters and cell towers, toxic inoculations, poor sleeping habits, and low sun exposure all make for a recipe for disaster.

You can understand the causes and make the necessary changes to restore your natural prostate health. The body can heal itself naturally if you eliminate the causes and nourish it with vital nutrients.

This is so obvious, it's worth repeating: Stop the causes, cleanse, modify your diet, and allow healing to occur by changing the internal conditions of the body!

Here's my list of causes for prostate cancer:

> How our constitution and conditions will impact us. This includes genes.

> Our diets--this is so major. Your medicine is food. Food is essential to your health. Bad food quality can lead to disease.

> Poor stress management: It is well-known that stress can have a negative impact on our health, and it may also affect our hormone balance by decreasing much-needed testosterone levels.

> Your lifestyle and inactivity--do nothing, and you will get something! We were created to move and not stay put.

> We need to get out of our sedentary lives. The prostate is irritated by sitting too long. Your prostate will be decongestible if you get up from your desk regularly and move around.

> Avoid harmful habits such as smoking and excessive alcohol consumption.

> Sugar intake is the main fuel source for most cancers. The most harmful form of fructose sugar, which is widely consumed today, disrupts leptin hormones and impacts testosterone levels. Sugar: The Bitter Truth

> Toxicity--toxic buildup (dioxins/bpa, herbicides) in the environment, personal care products, and commercial and GMO food has a significant impact on our health.

A new study has shown that Roundup herbicide, which is Monsanto's active ingredient, may be the most disruptive chemical in the environment. It can cause a variety of health disorders, including Parkinson's and cancer, as well as other diseases, such as autism and cancer.

> Too many wrong kinds of fats can lead to tumor formation. High levels of omega 6 vegetable fats can cause cancer. High levels of processed vegetable fats in modern times lower testosterone levels, which can lead to excessive estrogen. High estrogen and low testosterone are opposites of what a healthy person wants. . . These are the perfect conditions for prostate cancer.

Harvard University has released a new study that shows pasteurized milk products from factory farms can cause hormone-dependent cancers. The CAFO model of milk production from cows raised on factory farms produces dangerously high levels estrone. This estrogen compound is linked to breast, testicular and prostate cancers. Natural

This is the leading cause of prostate cancer. Northerly climates have fewer hours of sunlight and require more exposure. You are at risk of developing prostate cancer if you don't get enough vitamin D or sun exposure. Your risk of developing prostate cancer increases the further north you live. Vitamin D, also known as a hormone, is low in both black and white men. Black men are more likely to develop cancer than white men. This is due in part to their twice the rate of incidence of this disease compared with white American men, who have some of the highest rates of cancer worldwide. To build safe levels of Vitamin D, dark skin requires more sunlight.

> Insufficient oxygen--our cells lack oxygen because of pollution and inactivity.

> Vaccines, mercury fillings and too many antibiotics - these weaken the immune system and make us more vulnerable to diseases.

> Micro-waved and irradiated food--this unnatural heating method causes food to lose nutrients.

> Thyroid deficiencies increase the risk of developing cancer in significant ways. Read more: Dr. Michael Cutler

> Prostate cancer is often caused by hormone imbalances in men. Excess estrogen and hormonal imbalances can be caused by poor diets or plastic toxins that mimic estrogen.

Poor water quality and fluoride added to it can add toxins to an already overburdened immune system.

There are increasing reports about the harmful effects of electromagnetic fields (EMFs) from cell towers, smartphones, Wi-fi hubs, and smart meters on our immune system, and potential to cause cancer. Learn how to reduce exposures.

Poor sleep or not enough sleep. Long-term sleep problems or not enough sleep may make it twice as likely for men to get prostate cancer than those who sleep well. Why? Because testosterone levels are lower when you sleep less.

> Agri-foods grown in soils with low nutrients, which are unable to provide the crops the nutrients they require and the nutrients we need. The soil's vitality has declined dramatically since the advent of modern agriculture. A lack of essential nutrients can cause the body to be deficient in selenium, magnesium and other minerals which are vital for healthy prostates and high testosterone levels. When in reality, you think that healthy foods are nutritious, they can actually be harmful.

> Many household products and bodycare products can contain cancer-causing ingredients. Flame retardant chemicals are used on many carpets, furniture, and clothing. Excess estrogens can be caused by these chemicals, similar to BPA.

> Food additives, many which can be toxic:

The vast majority of chemical additives allowed in food, around 10,000, are supported only by safety assessments that have been funded and supported by the industry. This is according to new research published in JAMA Internal Medicine. A large number of these additives have not been submitted for review to the U.S. Food and Drug Administration, which means that the general population is being used as a collective guinea-pig in an enormous food additive safety experiment.

> 'Safety Assessments' on Nearly all Common Food Additives Found to be Manipulated by Processed Food Industry: Study by J. Benson, http://www.naturalnews.com/041703_safety_assessments_food_add itiv

> Side effects of some BPH (enlarged prostate medication) can cause prostate cancer. If you have an enlarged or swollen prostate, be sure to ask your doctor for advice. Finasteride, Proscar and Propecia, Dutasteride (Avodart), turosteride, bexlosteride and izonsteride-- significantly increases the risk of acquiring a fatal form of prostate cancer. These drugs can also be used to treat baldness, so men beware! For more information about Finasteride, click the link.

Look at this list, which Dr. Mercola has compiled - of 10 American Foods that have been banned in other countries - if you believe the FDA is trying to protect you.

> farmed salmon

> Genetically engineered papaya

> Ractopamine-tainted meat found in approximately 45% of American pigs

30% of ration-fed cattle and an unknown portion of turkeys

> flame-retardant drinks

> Processed foods that contain artificial food colours and dyes

> arsenic-laced chicken

> Bread with potassium bromate

> olestra/olean is a fat substitute that is calorie-, cholesterol- and fat-free. It can be used in fat-free snacks

> Preservatives BHA/BHT found in breakfast cereals, nut mixtures, chewing gum and butter spread.

> Milk and dairy products laced rBGH (Monsanto's growth hormone).

Are you concerned that any of these might contribute to prostate cancer. You have to take control of your health.

My book Healthy Prostate explains the risks and the ways in which modern medical treatments can spread prostate cancer. It also outlines the tests that may increase your chance of spreading it. My website also covers these topics. The best thing for prostate cancer patients is to wait patiently, as it can be fatal in well over 90% cases. If prostate cancer is not treated, men who are diagnosed with it will likely die from another form of cancer. These side effects, such as impotence, urinary and fecal problems, are avoided.

Learn more about the most recent insights on prostate cancer screening:

Medical Announcement: Prostate Cancer Is Almost All Failed to Tell You

PSA Screening - Complete Medical Hoax: 99.9% of the time it provides no benefit to men

Why should the after effects of some prostate cancer treatments be worse than the disease itself?

Quality of life is more important than quantity, so "watchful waiting" makes sense. However, you don't have to wait. Be proactive and empowered in your healthcare.

This takes effort! You will not get a solution from someone else. This proactive approach may not be for everyone. I urge men who desire real health, not a mere facsimile that could lead to you losing your ability have sex and control of your bladder, to expand their understanding. This is what I call Plan B.

Plan B is to understand the causes of prostate cancer. Then you can decide what course of action to take. You can see that you need to address the inputs you receive (everything you eat or drink, inhale, or absorb into your body).

Your diet should be improved if you want to fight prostate cancer. This will improve your overall health, and prevent your prostate cancer spreading.

This book can help you prevent prostate cancer. Learn what's next!

It is not rocket science. Stopping the causes is the only way to prevent or treat them. Eat real food. This means that you should replace pre-packaged, processed, factory food with healthy foods, foods similar to what we ate 100 year ago. Cleanse your body from any toxic buildup.

What should you do? Learn. Changes are possible. Day by day, one by one. Your health is yours, not the doctor's. Turn the page and learn.

Chapter 3: The Prostate Cancer Prevention Diet

Our health and well-being is determined by our food choices. Your health and the condition of your prostate are directly affected by your food choices. It can make us lose or gain health.

The Prostate Cancer Prevention Diet doesn't fit all. This diet focuses on your needs and the specifics of your body.

It is important that you realize that diet theory is not the same as reality. Expert pundit advice has often made my health worse.

Every book on diet and health that I've read and every doctor I've met seem to have very specific ideas about the ideal diet.

It is easy to believe that the food you eat or the diet you follow are the best. It's something you have studied and adopted. You are very invested in your choices, habits, and opinions.

Yes, I do! After a famous pundit's advice, I did it for 35 years! My method was perfect until I couldn't pee one night. Then I started following other experts.

I was able to work from home, where there was great air quality, water quality and good food. I also had the ability to easily implement healthy lifestyles without making compromises. It could be said that I was the ideal candidate to test various diets.

My prostate seemed to be getting worse. Their diet plans had many good aspects, so how could I have gotten worse rather than better?

Sometimes, I'd wake up in the middle of the night and have an unexpected shut down. No matter how much I wanted to urinate, I could not!

I began to realize that there were certain indulgences and deviations which could be very harmful for my prostate health. They could have a serious impact on my prostate health so I tried to avoid them as much as possible.

Two things were then revealed to me that gave me a great breakthrough:

> How to test if the food I am about to eat is healthy for me

> How to avoid common foods and prepare them to reduce a harmful anti-nutrient.

These breakthroughs were so profound, I felt a shift in my health. Finally, I began to recover.

Change is difficult for most people because they are used to their routines. However, in the case your prostate condition, the health and pain relief that comes with being healthy is well worth the effort.

The Prostate Cancer Prevention Diet, which is custom-made for you by yourself, is dynamically evolving in real time and based upon key principles that make perfect sense to you.

Consider the following potential benefits:

> You can avoid serious side effects of conventional medical options such as impotence and incontinence. These two were enough to motivate me, I don't know if you do too!

> Increase your overall health and well-being, which can increase your life span and make you live longer with less "what ails you?" as your age.

> Feel and look younger.

> Lose weight and feel great!

If you are forced to pay for traditional healthcare, save money. It is possible to save both time and money by avoiding costly procedures.

Now I will share with you what I believe is the best way to get on the path to good health.

Which is the Best Diet for You?

Isn't this the key question?

Every person is different. Each person's nutritional requirements will vary depending on their genetic inheritance, constitution, current health, and the toxic burden we have left behind over the course of our lives.

The ratios of needed nutrients from foods--carbohydrates, proteins and fats as well as the need for different vitamins and minerals--vary from person to person.

A diet that does not reflect our individuality, which is our biochemical uniqueness and overall health condition, is not the right one. For a few, it may be effective.

Before you begin tailoring your diet to suit you and your body, there are some things you should know. Let's start with the basics.

How the 20th Century Changed the West's Food

The West's agricultural practices have changed drastically over the past 20 years. They are now experiencing huge growth in the following:

> Hormones given to animals

> chemicals and contaminants in our water supplies

> Using grains as the primary input to increase milk production and meat production, which is an unnatural primary food for cows. This has unhealthy consequences for them and for us.

> Pasteurization and homogenization milk and dairy products

> Chemically produced vegetable oils

> Consumption of denatured grains such as white breads, cakes, and cookies

> Consumption of trans fats and hardened oils like margarine

> Sugar consumption as well as deadly artificial sugar intake

> Excessive medication and antibiotics

> harmful vaccines

> Fluoridation and Chlorination of Our Water Supplies

> Regular feeding of livestock by-products

> Bioconcentration of Toxins up the Food Chain

> Chemical fertilizer use, herbicides, and pesticides

> Factory farms are where animals are kept in small spaces and protected from serious diseases by antibiotics.

> Using city sewage (sludge), for fertilizer purposes in farms with high concentrations of toxic residues from all types of medical products and medical discards

> Using only a handful of seed types can reduce our food variety and decrease trace elements in a diverse food supply

> monoculture cropping methods that have depleted the soil's mineral content over the past century. This farming method uses petroleum-based chemical fertilizers, which deplete the soil of essential minerals like zinc, magnesium, and selenium. These vital minerals are critical for prostate health.

Genetically modified foods (GM) are now in nearly all of the soy, sugarbeet, and corn products we eat, as well as many commercial supplements.

These changes can have a negative impact on the quality of our food and denature it, which can lead to diseases, particularly when they are combined with Western lifestyle choices.

The key factor is time. Although one meal may not have an impact on the body, consuming a lot of these foods over time will eventually lead to chronic diseases, which are now epidemics in the West.

Food Manufacturing Practices

This list does not include food manufacturing practices that are more harmful than the ones mentioned above:

> Adding high fructose corn syrup to most prepared foods and soft beverages

> artificial sweeteners that are not properly metabolized and alien to the body

> MSG and its derivatives, such as hydrolyzed proteins, are carcinogenic.

> Adding all sorts of toxic chemicals and preservatives to our food

> removing the hulls from grain products to strip nutrients and make them "white".

> Significantly increasing sugar and salt content of our food

> artificial flavors and colors

> Using chemicals and high heat to make vegetable oils

> Using margarine and transfats in food preparation

This article explains the dangers of common ingredients in supermarket food: What's Really in the Food?

These are all things you know! It is possible that you have relied on your strong constitution to temporarily prevent disaster, or believed the medical symptomatic view that disease "happens" in the real world.

You can make this better, as I've said before. It is possible to avoid getting sick.

Slowly Toxins Become Your Enemy

Toxic overload of hormone-disrupting and estrogen-mimicking chemicals (known collectively as "xenoestrogens") can cause hormonal imbalance and lead to prostate problems.

It's no surprise that we have so many illnesses!

Hormone disruptors include pesticides, herbicides, and fungicides that are associated with non-organic foods, chemicals leached from plastic bottles and water from food can linings, and cleaners used in your home. They also include nonstick surfaces in pots and pans and chemically fireproofed mattresses.

Extremely high estrogen levels in men today can cause changes in testosterone levels, male breast development, and erectile dysfunction. One of the most common causes of prostate cancer is excessive estrogen.

Every man has some estrogen. An excess of estrogen can lead to a loss in the healthy testosterone-to-estrogen ratio. Trans fats, toxic foods, and estrogen mimicking chemicals are all factors that can cause this imbalance. . . ... and many more.

It is extremely frightening to have toxins in your body together. They can be deadly in combination by many orders of magnitude.

Men almost always develop prostate disease, including cancer, as they age.

Our bodies fight to survive when we eat so many foods that are laced with chemicals. It is not hard to understand why our prostate condition rates are so high.

It reminds me of a story about a frog that is placed in a pot filled with water. It should be heated slowly so that the frog does not die!

How can we stop these causes? You can reduce the toxic effects and increase food quality and cleansing. It is possible to reverse the damage done over the years or reduce the severity of the disease. For men to be healthy, they need to eat natural foods and get Vitamin D from the sun.

BPA

Bisphenol A can be found in the cans that your canned food is stored in, as well as in plastics used to make water. You are exposed to even more toxins.

BPA mimics estrogen and is an endocrine disruptor. It can cause imbalanced hormone levels, and lower testosterone.

We can add toxic substances to our diet, whether we know it or not.

Our prostate is automatically stressed and toxins are deposited into it. One day, suddenly, prostate disease strikes. Now you understand the true cause and the obvious solution: Change your inputs!

Neurotoxins

Many processed and restaurant food items are laced with neurotoxins as flavor enhancers. This applies to many healthy-sounding chemicals, as well as organic ones.

Neurotoxins are absorbed from nerve endings and travel within the neuron to the cell bodies, disrupting vital functions.

These ingredients can cause severe health reactions and weight gain, as well as cancers. It is important to learn how to read labels. You can find dangerous, artificial additives in both packaged and restaurant-prepared food.

MSG.

The most well-known neuro-toxins is monosodium glutamate, (MSG). These protein additives can be called many different names. . . Even "natural flavors", a pleasant-sounding term, can be a sign that there are toxic additives to the brain or nervous system.

. . .

Spikes is a sign that toxic additives may be hidden in the product. . . You can't know the answer unless you take the time to read each label.

The Packaged and Hidden Health Saving Neurotoxins contain a Hundred of Health-Sapping Neurotoxins

Restaurant Food by B. L. Minton

www.naturalnews.com/026244_food_MSG_neurotoxins.html

Here are some other neurotoxic chemical food additives:

> aspartame Nutrasweet

> beef flavoring

> protein concentrate

> bouillon protein extract

> salt seasoned with caseinate

> Chicken flavoring seasoning

> smoke flavoring

> glutamate soy extract

> hydrolyzed ingredients

> soy protein

> corn protein

> wheat protein

> Milk solids spice

> monosodium glutamate

> Textured vegetable protein

> natural flavor

> yeast extract

It is a good idea to read labels before you buy food!

Pesticides

Pesticides found in food can be powerful endocrine disruptors. They directly impact our hormones. Men are affected by pesticides in their food. They increase the production of estrogens in the females and weaken their prostate glands, which rely on healthy levels testosterone.

Pesticides can also impact your mood and body weight, as well as your chances of developing prostate cancer. It's no wonder that so few couples can conceive naturally today!

The average American consumes over a gallon each year of pesticides, and other health-threatening chemicals. Even though many toxic chemicals are eliminated, eventually our immune system is compromised. These toxins are absorbed by fat tissue and can cause weight gain or the onset chronic health conditions.

We now know who the enemy is, from government to agribiz and mass processed food producers, fast food chains to our supermarkets or restaurants, and finally, us who eat them! We are our worst enemy!

The Environmental Working Group (EWG), analyzed the pesticide residues on 47 fruits, vegetables, and 87,000 test results were taken between 2000 and 2007. This resulted in a classification of toxic and most contaminated produce. EWG's Shopper's Guide contains more information about pesticides in fruits and vegetables.

Here's a list with the most harmful pesticide foods - the higher the number, then the food is considered to be dangerous:

peach	100
apple	93
sweet bell pepper	83
celery	82
nectarine	81
strawberries	80
cherries	73
kale	69
lettuce	67
grapes (imported)	66
carrots	63
pear	63
collard greens	60
spinach	58
potatoes	56
green beans	53
summer squash	53
pepper	51
cucumber	50
raspberries	46
grapes (domestic)	44
plums	44
oranges	44
cauliflower	39
tangerines	37
mushrooms	36

bananas	34
winter squash	34
cantaloupe	33
cranberries	33
honeydew melon	30
grapefruit	29
sweet potatoes	29
tomatoes	29
broccoli	28
watermelon	26
papaya	20
eggplant	20
cabbage	17
kiwi	13
sweet peas (frozen)	10
asparagus	10
mango	9
pineapple	7
sweet corn (frozen)	2
avocado	1
onion	1

Note. 100 = the worst pesticide load. 1 = the least pesticide load.

It is best to switch to organic versions for anything above 25. You could also use the other varieties if you needed to, but they would still be low in nutrients due to the soils that they were grown on. While non-organic produce might look beautiful, it lacks selenium as well as a host other essential minerals for your health.

Genetically Modified Foods

Several countries around the globe have banned genetically modified or genetically engineered food. You can find the American Academy of Environmental Medicine's warning here to avoid genetically modified food.

No one knows what the consequences are of inserting new genes into a product and then eating it for many generations. We know that food-related illnesses doubled when GMO's were introduced to the market. GMO foods are:

> Allergenic

> Toxic

> Carcinogenic

> Anti-nutritional

Roundup herbicide has been linked with a host of physiological problems, including birth defects, the destruction and loss of testosterone, and male fertility. Two scientists have published Entropy in peer-reviewed journal. They claim that glyphosate (the active ingredient in Monsanto's Roundup herbicide) is responsible for many health conditions and diseases, including Parkinson's and cancer.

Dr. Mercola makes a remarkable comparison between the nutritional value of GM and non-GM corn:

According to a report by an employee at Dell Seed Company, Canada's only non GMO corn seed company, genetic modification is making modern food less nutritious. This amazing picture shows the nutritional differences between non-GM and genetically modified corn. The former is clearly not equivalent to the latter. This is the very basis on which genetically modified crops were approved. This 2012 nutritional analysis shows just a few of the nutritional differences:

> Calcium: GMO corn = 14 ppm Non-GMO corn = 6,130 ppm (437 times more)

> Magnesium: GMO Corn = 2 ppm Non GMO corn = 113ppm

(56 times more)

> Manganese: GMO corn = 2 ppm   Non-GMO corn = 14 ppm (7 times more)

Breeding the Nutrition Out of Our Food by Dr. Mercola, http://articles.mercola.com/sites/articles/archive/2013/06/11/modernfood-nutritional-content.aspx?

Jeffrey Smith's book, Seeds of Deception: Exposing Government and Industry Lies about the Safety of Genetically Engineered Foods You Eat, provides a detailed education on the dangers of GM food.

You can read more about Roundup and birth defects in these articles: Roundup: Are we keeping the public ignorant? Study: Roundup diluted by 99.8 per cent still damages human DNA.

This site provides more information about the effects of animal kidneys and livers.

An Anatomical Record published 2009 findings on significant changes in the reproductive cycles and uterus of rats. A French study published in 2009 in the International Journal of Biological Sciences revealed long-term effects of Monsanto corn fertilizer Roundup on rats. The rats suffered from grotesque tumors, organ damage, and early death.

Continue reading about Irina Eramkova's study at the Russian National Academy of Sciences on mother rats that were fed GM soybeans: GM Soy Dangerous for Newborns?

GMO-free foods are being banned in many countries.

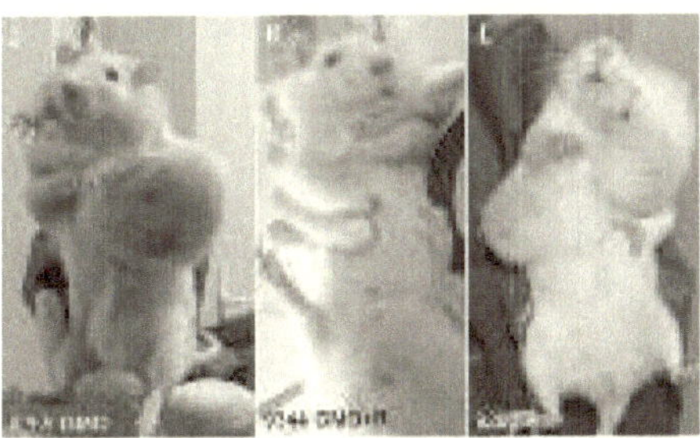

Reprinted from Food and Chemical Toxicology 50(11), Seralini G.

Clair E., Mesnage, R., Gress, S., Defarge, N., Malatesta, M.,

Hennequin (D.) & de Vendomois (J. S.). Long-Term Toxicity of Roundup Pesticides and Roundup-tolerant Genetically Modified maize. Copyright (2012) with permission from Elsevier.

Avoid processed foods as they may contain up to 70% GM food. Soy and corn are found in the majority of processed and fast-food products!

The Institute for Responsible Technology has published the Non-GMO Shopping Guide.

Vitamins & Minerals

Chapter 9 focuses on how to get the vitamins and minerals you need from food sources. I also discuss when to take pills to supplement your diet. This chapter should not be rushed. Next, I will discuss deficiency and depletion as well as anti-nutrients.

Modern agricultural practices have led to major depletion of vital vitamins and minerals in our food, as well as major deficiencies in essential trace minerals. Modern food processing adds to the problem by increasing anti-nutrients. Vitamin and mineral deficiencies are another major cause of illness.

Depletion

Let's look at the extent to which modern commercial farming has reduced our food supply. The U.S. Department of Agriculture has compiled a list of the nutritional value of fruits and vegetables in comparison to 1975:

Fruit or Vegetable	Nutritional Value Change since 1975
Apples	Vitamin A is down 41%
Sweet Peppers	Vitamin C is down 31%
Watercress	Iron is down 88%
Broccoli	Calcium and Vitamin A are down 50%
Cauliflower	Vitamin C is down 45%; Vitamin B1 is down 48%; Vitamin B2 is down 47%
Collards Greens	Vitamin A is down 45%; Potassium is down 60%; Magnesium is down 85%

Wow! Wow.

Deficiency

Consuming conventional food is a fast way to deprive your body of vital nutrients. Organic foods have grown at a compound rate 25% per annum for over a decade. Many people are now realizing that conventional food has a detrimental effect on their health and the cost of organic foods is too high.

Your body's proper functioning depends on trace minerals such as zinc and selenium. Yet, almost all trace minerals are greatly depleted in soils that produce our food.

This is because conventional agriculture takes these minerals out of the soils year after year and then doesn't replenish them.

Conventional fertilizers have virtually no trace minerals. This means that after only a decade of conventional farming, soils have become depleted in essential trace minerals your body requires to function. Conventional agriculture is almost like strip mining. It takes valuable minerals from the soil and transports them in the food, eventually leaving the soils depleted.

Why You Should Get Your Selenium and Zinc from Foods, Not Synthetic Vitamins by M. Adams,
www.naturalnews.com/031397_MegaFood_zinc.html

This book will prove that you are wrong if you believe taking a mineral supplement will solve your problem.

Anti-Nutrients

An anti-nutrient can be a synthetic or natural compound that hinders your body's ability to absorb vitamins, minerals, or other nutrients. The most important for prostate health is phytic Acid.

What is Phytic Acid?

A variety of foods contain the antinutrient phytic acids, also known as phytotates. Whole grains, beans, pulses nuts, seeds, and whole grains all contain phytic acid. This helps plants protect themselves against insect predators and prevents premature germination. These seeds can be stored for a long period of time because they contain phytic acid.

These foods make up a lot of modern food, but they are often poorly prepared, such as packaged cereals, breads, and their whole-grain versions, rice cakes and soups, and other soy additives. These foods are available in fast food restaurants and supermarkets.

Unfortunately, phytic acid can cause irritation in the body and gradually remove vital minerals. Phytic acid is a phytic acid that binds to calcium, iron and zinc, and slowly removes them from your body.

These minerals are essential for healthy and vibrant health. A lack of them can lead to all kinds of health problems later in life. These elements are subject to a cumulative reduction over time.

Zinc deficiencies can be a problem in the male reproductive system. The prostate needs a lot of zinc for proper functioning.

Zinc is essential for good health.

Reduced calcium levels can also lead to osteoporosis and cavities. Low levels of magnesium can lead to many diseases. See Magnesium Is Vital for Good Health for more information.

Magnesium is a vital mineral that our bodies need, especially in these times when we are exposed to so many toxins and heavy metals on a daily basis. Our bodies will age faster and degenerate if we accumulate toxins and acid residues. Magnesium is essential for our cells' survival.

This mineral is essential for the prevention of cancer. This mineral is extremely potent and can prevent the calcification of tissues and organs.

Research is proving the health benefits of magnesium as both a detox method and a key component in natural cancer treatment. Magnesium can be added to most foods. A simple spray on the skin that is water-based can be used to increase magnesium intake. This is a cost-effective and efficient way to get more magnesium.

Magnesium protects cells from lead, mercury, cadmium and beryllium. This explains why remineralization is essential for heavy metal detoxification, chelation, and radiation protection. Magnesium is vital for our survival, but it becomes even more important when our bodies are bombarded daily with heavy metals or radiation.

Magnesium Offers Strong Radiation Protection by M. Sircus, www.naturalnews.com/032596_magnesium_radiation.html

You can find more information about magnesium at Dr. Sircus' blog-- Magnesium oil. Beans are a good source of magnesium.

(black and kidney), green veggies (broccoli, spinach), seafood (oysters rockfish, rockfish and scallops), nuts (sesame and flax), cashews (pumpkin and squash seeds), lentils (rice, oats, wheat), chocolate, molasses, and herbs.

A 15-20 minute soak in Epsom salts helps to absorb magnesium through the skin.

The adverse effects of phytates found in food are also detrimental. They can cause digestive problems. Phytic acid blocks enzymes that aid digestion, including amylase to convert starch into sugar, pepsin to break down stomach proteins and amylase to turn starch into glucose.

Download a complete article on phytates: Cereal Grains: Humanity's Double-Edged Sword.

Properly prepared food is essential. Even "healthy" foods need to be properly prepared in order to ensure proper digestion and the removal of any depletion that may cause anti-nutrients. Proper preparation was a key component of the whole food-natural foods revolution, which began in the 1970s. Many foods found in health food stores today aren't healthy due to poor preparation!

This article, Living with Phytic Acid, provides a detailed article about phytic acid and its reduction techniques.

Phytic Acid Levels in Some Foods

Below is a list of foods that contain the anti-nutrient phytotic acid (phytates). These foods should not be avoided, but we need to learn how to get rid of phytates using traditional food preparation methods. We risk developing undiagnosed diseases over time.

Fermenting or soaking are the best ways to reduce phytates. However, sprouting and sourdough leavingning can also be helpful. If phytate-rich foods do not get soaked first they will remain in the food.

Puffed grains and cereal flakes are two of the worst culprits. These supposed healthy cereals are now deadly because of the highheat extrusion process. Cardboard is healthier than Breakfast Cereal.

Start changing your cooking habits by using these foods as a preventative measure:

Food	Phytic Acid (mg/100g)

Sesame seeds dehulled	5,360
100% Wheat bran cereal	3,290
Soybeans	1,000–2,220
Cocoa powder	1,684–1,796
Oats	1,370
Brown rice	1,250
Oat flakes	1,174
Coconut meal	1,170
Almonds	1,138–1,400
Parboiled brown rice	1,600
Barley	1,190
Whole corn	1,050
Rye	1,010
Walnut	982
Whole wheat flour	960
Lentils	779
Navy beans	740–1,780
Hazelnuts	648–1,000
Wild rice flour	634–753
Refried beans	622
Peanuts germinated	610
Pinto beans	600–2,380
Corn tortillas	448

Corn	367
White flour	258
White flour tortillas	123

Note. Note: Measurements are expressed in milligrams for every 100 grams of weight. Source: (Part

I) Whole Grain Toxicity - Phytic Acid Contained In Popular Foods The Weston A. Price Foundation documents:

Researchers often fail to realize that seeds foods, which include grains, legumes, and nuts, are prepared in traditional societies with care. They are soaked, sprouted, roasted, steamed, fermented, and sour leftned. These methods neutralize certain substances in whole grains and other seeds foods, which can block mineral absorption, hinder protein digestion, and irritate your digestive tract lining. These processes increase the nutritional content of seed foods and make them more digestible.

Are you naive, brutish and short? S. F. Morell

www.westonaprice.org/traditional-diets/nasty-brutish-short

You can learn more about phytates here and get great recipes at Rebuild Market--Phytic acid Drill-Down.

If these phytate-rich foods are not prepared correctly, they can cause sudden, unexplained prostate attacks (e.g. blockages, frequent urination, and more). I believe that phytates play a major role in the enlargement of prostates and other diseases. This is especially true when combined with poor eating habits and depleted commercially toxic foods.

Nourishing Traditions is a great book. This book will teach you the how and why of good food preparation. This book is full of delicious recipes, important information about diets and phytate-reducing tips.

If you are unsure of how to cook your meals or if I have a lot to say that is new, please do not hesitate to purchase the book. There are tons of great recipes!

Another great resource for information and tips is Phytic Acid-Tips For Consumers From Food Science.

This is a detailed explanation of phytic acids in foods. Although the source comes from a Paleo diet perspective (which I have reservations about as discussed later), this article is a great insight into some of the dangers associated with eating healthy foods. Find out What's Wrong With Beans and Legumes.

Prepare Your Food with Traditional, Time-Tested Methods

As long as you are healthy, small amounts of phytate rich foods daily may not cause harm. However, sensitive people will experience reactions. Large amounts of phytate-rich foods over time can lead to severe health problems.

There are many ways to prepare your grains, beans and pulses so that the phytic acid level is reduced.

To reduce the harmful effects of anti-nutrients on your body, soak foods. To further reduce the phytates, you can sprout them or add sea salt to them.

This chart is very useful for this purpose. Drag it to your desktop, and then print: Whole Food Lab Soak & Sprout.

Soak nuts in warm water. Use lukewarm water to dissolve the sea salt. Leave the nuts to soak overnight. Rinse and dry the nuts at 150°F until they become crunchy. For this, I use my toaster oven.

Grain soak overnight for best results. Rinse, then cook. Soaked foods cook faster.

Beans do best soaked for longer periods (12-24 hours), and then rinsed in warm water. Rinse well and then cook. You can also add some kombu seaweed to aid digestion. These steps not only reduce harmful elements, but also increase the body's absorption of minerals and nutrients.

After I began personal testing (see Chapter 10) I realized how wrong my assumption that I had a healthy diet consisting of vegetables, fruits, nuts, seeds, and grains was. Anti-nutrients such as phytic acid are what I now know caused my severe prostate reactions. It was very difficult for me to admit that I had been wrong for 35+ years. It was time to question my assumptions and examine the best foods for me at each moment. It was also very empowering to finally find the answers to my prostate problem!

Eat According to Your Local Climate

You should eat according to the season, your climate, and environment. Your body will adjust to the climate by producing vitamin D. This ensures that your body is able to digest food properly.

Modern conveniences of cooling and transport allow us to eat foods out of season, but eating food from different climates or zones can cause problems with our digestive systems and disrupt our hormones. This is not something you want for your prostate!

Local food is the best. Sunlight is good for your skin. Avoid eating raw foods and avoid tropical foods if you are unable to get the sun. Why? Because the sun tells our bodies that fresh, seasonal food is good to eat.

You will end up eating foods that will harm your health if you don't pay attention to your climate and the food that is best for you there.

Raw foods can be delicious for a brief time in hot climates, but think about eating bananas and watermelons in Alaska during a January deep freeze! You will be fine if you are only enjoying it as a treat. But if you eat raw fruits and vegetables regularly, your body will eventually suffer.

Sounds drastic, doesn't it? All of this is easy to understand once you learn about the ileocecal valv. The ileocecal valve lies between the large intestine and the small intestine. It prevents the flora from your large intestine backing up into your small intestine, where it can cause havoc.

Your ileocecal valve can be damaged by eating the wrong foods, in the wrong climate, and at the wrong times of the year. This valve requires calcium, magnesium, and vitamin D from your body to stay strong.

Your body will not produce vitamin D if it is exposed to foods from other countries or foods out of season. Why? Potassium is found in all plant-derived foods. Higher levels of potassium are found in tropical plant-based foods. They are higher in potassium than we consume. Our kidneys detect the higher potassium levels and assume that we are living in a sunny area with lots of vitamin D!

You'll suddenly have trouble with your digestion. This is something you might not notice, but it depends on many factors. Watch out for digestive problems! Bad bacteria can cause liver damage, which in turn can lead to digestive problems and eventually, a poor health. This can lead to food reactions, irritable stool, and other problems in your prostate, including inability to properly deploy hormones.

Dr. Jonn Matsen is a world-class Naturopathic Doctor who has written an insightful book about the many chronic health issues that plague our modern society.

His simple message is:

You could easily lose your sanity if you don't spend enough time out in the sun.

Calcium absorption--and in five days your ileocecal valve might be weak enough for your billions worth of good bacteria to flood into your small intestine.

The Yeast Are Back by J. Matsen, www.eatingalive.com/march2012the-yeast-are-back/

Even the best quality food can make your condition worse or delay your healing. This is a very important point to remember!

He suggested that he stop eating raw foods for six days. Sea salt is a high-quality ingredient that can be added to lightly cooked vegetables. He recommends that you take a high-quality vitamin D and calcium supplement: Cal Mag liquid, and this for your liver: SC Liver Formula.

You will be amazed at the results of the 6-day test. You will be amazed! I was.

You can then begin his program to eliminate yeast overgrowth. You will be amazed at the impact it has on your health. Bio-Nutritional Formulas-- Latero Flora Powder

Start with 1/4 teaspoon of yeast every three days. Then increase it to 1/8th teaspoon. It is best not to rush yeast kill. This can cause liver damage. Adjust accordingly and take it slow.

His book explains everything you need to know and why. The book is illustrated with simple cartoon diagrams, which simplify complicated issues and make them easy to comprehend.

He has treated thousands of patients with amazing results. He's well-known for his ability to "cure the incurable." He's a warm, friendly, and affordable doctor.

His talk on the dangers associated with amalgam fillings is as world-class as his views on vaccines.

This book, Eating Alive II is a must-read if you have mercury fillings and/or aren't making any progress with your healing.

Unseasonal, nonlocal eating can lead to long-term health problems and weight gain. You are vulnerable to side effects that can be minor or major if your digestion is not optimal.

It is easier to digest cooked vegetables than raw foods, especially in winter. Be local and smart about what you eat. This can be easily tested by comparing the responses to cooked and raw foods. Learn more about personal testing in Chapter 10.

Continue reading to find out more about vitamin D, sunlight, and other aspects of vitamin D.

Sunlight Exposure

Insufficient sunlight is a major cause of prostate cancer. Northerly climates have shorter sunlight hours, so more exposure is required. Vitamin D, which is the most important nutrient to good health, acts as a hormone in your body.

Vitamin D research shows that the majority of people are not getting enough vitamin D. This means that you have a lower chance of developing cancer, especially prostate cancer, if your body has more vitamin D!

Modern Western men have a low level of vitamin D, particularly black and darker-skinned Americans whose skin was developed to withstand a lot of sun exposure. Black Americans are at highest risk for prostate cancer. Low levels of vitamin D are often linked to this risk.

Due to the lack of sunlight exposure, many Americans are severely deficient in vitamin-D during winter. Even those who live in sunny areas but spend too much indoors can also be severely deficient.

Sun exposure has been a fact of life for many. People now avoid the sun, use sunscreens that are toxic and can cause cancer, or cover up when they do.

There is overwhelming evidence that sun exposure has many benefits. Sun exposure that is responsible, meaning you avoid the most damaging midday sunrays, can be so beneficial. You should not use sunscreen for more than 15-20 minutes each day. This is the best form of sunscreen.

Start slowly if you have sensitive skin. Then, increase the volume until you cover at least 20 minutes of your body, ideally including your prostate. Nudist colonies have something to offer!

Your skin color will determine how dark you should apply sunscreen.

Because sun exposure is so important for your health, I encourage you to learn more about it. There are many good resources for information about vitamin D and sunlight:

"Vitamin D" is the most powerful medicine against cancer. It far surpasses the benefits of any other cancer drug.

Vitamin D and sunlight have healing benefits

The Sunscreen Myth: How Sunscreen Products Really Promote Cancer

"Epidemics" of Vitamin D Deficiency: MUHC Study

To reduce cancer risk, we need to consume more Vitamin D

If you're not convinced, read this extensive information from Vitamin D Council.

Supplementing with sardines and potent cod liver oils is the best way to get sunlight exposure if you don't have the time or can't go out on sunny days. (See Chapter 9 Cod Liver Oil). You are getting vitamin D directly from food sources rather than from a supplement.

Natural vitamin D3 supplements are the next best option for vitamin D, but they are not as effective as cod liver oil which has been tested over thousands of years. Refer to Chapter 9 for more information on Vitamin D.

Exercise

Anyone who speaks about health and nutrition must encourage readers to exercise. This is a crucial component to restoring your health or maintaining good health.

Weight training helps raise your testosterone levels. Because of the estrogen-rich foods and other toxins men have accumulated, this is a very important step in preventing prostate cancer.

You can't lose weight if you don't rev up your metabolism.

To increase quality and longevity in your life, exercise is essential. Sedentary lifestyles have a direct impact on the prostate. Your prostate will be happy if you get up and move around throughout the day!

Our bodies were made to move every day. For weight loss and other health benefits, we all know the importance of exercising.

It shouldn't be surprising, but it's always nice to hear this from professionals! Recent research on prostate cancer in men was done by the Harvard School of Public Health, and the University of California. This is the first time men with prostate cancer have been studied in order to determine their activity levels after being diagnosed and to then link it to mortality related to the cancer or general mortality.

It was found that exercise is associated with a lower death rate from prostate cancer and death all around. Men with prostate cancer who exercised more had a lower chance of dying. Stacey Kenfield, the Harvard School's lead author, stated that

The results of our study show that physical activity can help men reduce the risk of developing prostate cancer after being diagnosed. This is great news for prostate cancer patients who are unsure of the best lifestyle choices to increase their chances of survival.

These are the tips I've learned over years of being involved in these sports: swimming, biking, hiking and mountaineering; climbing and skiing. High intensity interval training (or strength training) can give you faster results than you might think.

Tips

> Do something that you love.

> Body exercises can help you get in shape for any sport (that are done with your own weight and not dumb dumbbells). Examples include push-ups and pull-ups, squats, lunges and skipping.

It is important to learn how to properly breathe while moving. You should breathe in and out through the nose and not your mouth. You can make the out-breath more powerful by drawing your stomach in simultaneously.

Training with intense bursts is much more effective than steady pacing. It also saves time. Only 10 minutes will do it!

> Perform 5-10 30-second bursts at high intensity, depending on your level. Start by walking. After warming up, slow down for 10 seconds

and then walk fast for another 1-2 minutes. Your heart rate and breath will return to normal. Continue this process several times. You can do 30 second bursts. Similar for swimming or running.

Variable routines can prevent injuries.

Stretching is also a great way to avoid injury.

Exercise can be fun if you do it for a reason.

Conclusion

Men with prostate problems are most often caused by modern factory-manufactured foods, toxicity, vitamin, mineral deficiencies, and lack of sunlight.

It's time to go back to our roots. It is time to make healthier living a priority and eat less.

Real food is more expensive . . But it may actually save you money. Many people have come to realize that conventional food has a high price and can have a negative impact on their health.

It is simple: Food can be either your medicine or poison.

Read on if you want to make food your medicine. Chapter 4 will give you an overview of the changes you can make in your diet.

Chapter 4: Healthy Eating Levels

This section provides a list of ideal and optimal diets, from the least healthy to the most nutritious. This scale provides a baseline to determine where your diet ranks, and also a guideline for changing your diet step-by-step.

Although you may feel that I am going too far, in reality we have gone too far in our food production choices and diet choices. Many of you may find my proposal too extreme because of modern lifestyles that have severely impacted our health.

Many people believe that they eat healthy food. If this is true why are there so many prostate diseases and poor quality of life as we get older?

Why is it that so many seniors are dependent on drugs and unhealthy? We are not vitally important until our old age?

In cultures that eat traditional, natural foods, prostate diseases are very rare. According to the medical profession, poor prostate health is due to the fact that we live longer. The cause is actually the accumulation of toxic substances from modern, devitalized non-foods, manufactured food concoctions, and poor food preparation.

You may come across so-called food experts when you are trying to eat healthier. I have repeatedly said that nobody can tell you what is best for you, only you.

One diet might recommend certain foods that are harmful to one body. However, there may be foods that the diet suggests you avoid that could be beneficial for another. No matter how scientific a diet is, we are all very different.

California is the fad capital of America, and many of the new diets are based there. For someone living in hot, sunny California, a raw diet may prove fatal for someone else. This is what the problem is with diet gurus, who claim that their way of eating is the best.

You can alter the way you eat and create a diet that suits your body. You may be sensitive to certain foods or reacting to them if you're undergoing a transition from a chronic condition. Don't despair! You will find that you can eat more if your health and condition improves.

These levels of healthy eating offer ideas for how to move up and change your diet at a time that suits you.

Poorest Diet

> Artificial sweeteners of any kind, such as Aspartame and Splenda (NutraSweet), and their products like diet soft drink

> beverages and foods sweetened by fructose, high fructose corn syrup or its derivatives

> Foods containing MSG, preservatives and other neurotoxic ingredients

> Highly processed, factory-made foods

> Foods containing growth hormones or antibiotics such as non-organic milk and meats

> Foods sprayed with pesticides

> GMO (Genetically Modified Organisms), foods that are foreign to the body (90% soy and corn, and their products in America contain GMOs). . . They are also fed to animals you eat.

> Food with vegetable trans fats

> Commercially manufactured vegetable oils and margarines

> Artificial food and food dyes

> meat from animals who are regularly fed grains, not grasses- and animal parts--and are raised in animal factories or a Concentrated Animal Feeding Operation.

> Grilled food (burnt fat, charred meat can cause cancer)

Yikes! How can we possibly be healthy if we eat such unhealthy foods? This is not a diet for prostate health.

Poor Diet

> commercially sprayed crops (vegetables, fruit)

> Refined carbs such as white flours and sugars are often laced in preservatives

> Undiscovered molds in manufactured food that are hidden behind preservatives

> Unripe fruits sprayed pesticides

> animal fats for commercial use

> fowl and meat grown in cramped quarters, fed antibiotic-laden feed such as grains and forage instead of grasses or forage.

> pasteurized and homogenized milk and dairy products

> High fructose corn syrup (and its products)

> Desserts with sugary and unhealthy fats

> canned food in BPA-lined containers

> table salt
> microwaved food
> margarine and oils that are partially or fully hydrogenated

> Preservatives are often used in processed meats and smoked meats. Hot dogs, deli meats, and hot dogs all contain preservatives.

> Commercial fast food

> Highly manufactured, packaged food with many ingredient >
Rice cakes, puffed cereals, etc.

These foods should be avoided at all costs. Take a look at the epidemic of diseases we have--from heart disease to diabetes, cancer, chronic illness, obesity, and degenerative diseases. These major diseases and problems are largely attributable to fast food and commercial food.

Acceptable Diet

> Fresh food but no commercial meat, dairy, or soy foods

> Minimal processed and packaged supermarket food

> Use butter and coconut oil instead of commercial vegetable oils or margarines.

> home cooked meals using fresh ingredients

> Free range fowl and free range meat

> frozen seafood

> No microwaved food

> Avoid GMO food and ingredients

> Restaurant food that isn't of fast food quality and is prepared with GMOfree natural products.

Good Food

> Organic produce and dairy

> Fresh seasonal local food

> fresh raw food

> seafood low in toxic metal fish

> Free-range meat and fowl

> Natural whole foods: Grains, beans, **seeds and nuts**

> sea salt

Organic restaurant food only

Optimum Food

> Home-grown and locally grown **fresh organic fruits & vegetables**

> Organic wild berries

> Real superfoods are a part of your **diet**

> Fresh organic raw food, sprouts (in moderation), and raw fermented vegetables

> healthy food for your body

> Non-pasteurized, raw organic milk from grass-fed animals

> Organic pasture-grazed, grass fed meat and fowl (not grains fed)

> Fresh-caught seafood and shellfish have the lowest toxic metal content

> Organic whole foods: Beans, seeds, grains, and nuts that have been soaked to lower phytic acid and other harmful nutrients

> Fresh wild foods and herbs

These lists highlight the differences in our food choices. Although it can be difficult to get up the food scale, it is an important choice to make if you want prostate health.

Eating well will ultimately be the best decision for your health.

You can choose to eat food that kills or nourishes you.

Conclusion

Food is complex. As you progress up the food pyramid, you will want to be able customize your diet to suit your needs and not just rely on theories. It is important to be able to determine what your body needs.

There is no perfect diet. No matter what food experts, including myself, may say, it doesn't matter. Your uniqueness is what makes you different.

When it comes to knowing the best foods for you, you are the master. However, "knowing" means learning and tuning in to your body. Your subconscious mind is the one who knows. Chapter 10 will give you a tool called personal testing that will allow you to tune inwards and see what is good for you right now. It's a simple, yet powerful tool.

In Chapter 5, I discuss the most current diets and show you why you should personalize your diet.

Chapter 5: Popular Diets

I will be discussing many popular diets and their pros and cons. But before I get into specific diets, I want you to consider two types of diets that are often misunderstood by many pundits: cleansing diets and nourishing diets.

Although cleansing diets can be used to remove toxins from the body, they are not recommended for long-term use. It should be used to accelerate the elimination of toxins and debris that has accumulated in your tissues and organs. It can cause problems if you keep a cleansing diet too long, especially if it isn't called a cleanse but a way to eat every day.).

These diets stimulate a strong immune response that helps to eliminate bad stuff. If we continue to do this for too long, our bodies become stressed and can develop new problems. Be sure to determine if you are undertaking a cleansing program. Also, keep in mind that there may be diminishing returns and other long-term risks.

One good example is a juice cleanse that contains fresh, raw fruit and vegetables. While it may work temporarily, long-term, it can be dangerous. As you'll soon see, raw food diets are harmful.

A healthy diet that is nourishing is the best for your long-term health. It must be based on solid principles and contain nutrients that your body can absorb easily. You will need to test different foods to make sure they are compatible with your particular condition.

This diet adapts to changing seasons, your location and your needs. It also uses the finest ingredients and preparation methods.

SAD—The Standard American Diet

It's sad. It is SAD. Many health advocates claim that the Standard American Diet is responsible for our epidemic of chronic diseases.

Jayson and Mira Calton, authors of Rich Food, Poor Food, claimed that ingredients found in as many as 80% of pre-packaged foods sold in the U.S. grocery stores have been banned in countries other than the United States.

We allow ourselves to be fooled into thinking that the fastest and cheapest food is acceptable to eat. There are no consequences to living this lifestyle, which includes C.R.A.P., caffeine, refined sugars and alcohol.

There are also hormones, antibiotics, fear-based hormones and hormones in the meat. We have toxic chemical fertilizers on our crops and our vegetables. Men with low sperm counts and infants born with inherited chemicals. Breast milk is unsafe and toxic for our babies.

Our government agencies do not protect us. They are a conduit for special interests groups that place the financial well-being of corporations above human safety.

We have accepted the advice of the media, agencies, and businesses to eat well. We ignore the evidence around us and shirk our responsibility to our health.

Our health has been deteriorating to the point that it is threatening our country and killing us. Government funds are used to pay for chronic diseases that could be avoided if we made healthy and conscious choices. When you examine the ingredients of many of these so-called healthy choices, you will find that they are often a deception.

Unfortunately, the Sick American Diet has replaced our Standard American Diet. This is why we have such high rates of chronic diseases. You can take pills, get irradiated or have surgery to continue your destructive patterns. But that is a joke.

Real treatment must address the root cause of the problem. Otherwise, it's just temporary relief to mask the symptoms.

Our ignorance is the root cause of prostate disease and all other chronic health issues. Unfortunately, this ignorance is not bliss. A loss of vibrancy is replacing vitality, which can lead to a life that is pain-free and fully functioning until old age.

You can learn and put an end to your SAD. That is the great news. Each day we make small changes. We choose the best foods and products for our health and we STOP, CLEANSE, and REVITALIZE.

Every person needs to be aware of their choices and take responsibility for their own care. These are some of the suggestions in The Prostate Cancer Prevention Diet. They promise a new and healthier you.

USDA Diet

The obesity rate has risen dramatically since 1980 when the U.S. Department of Agriculture released their food pyramid.

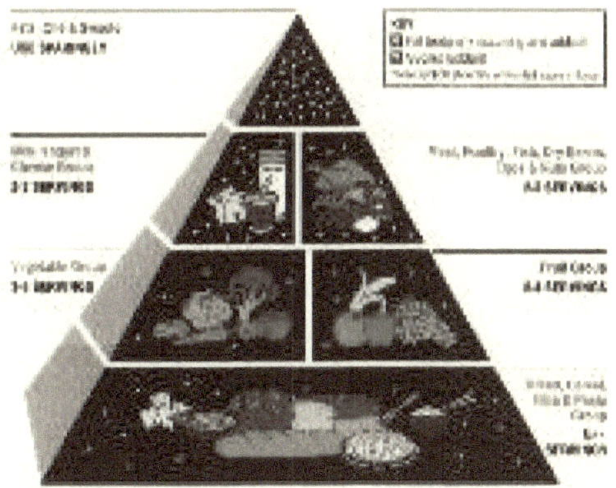

Source: U.S. Government, 1992. Food Pyramid.
http://en.wikipedia.org/wiki/Food_guide_pyramid

As you can see, the U.S. government changed their food pyramid to MyPlate in 2011.

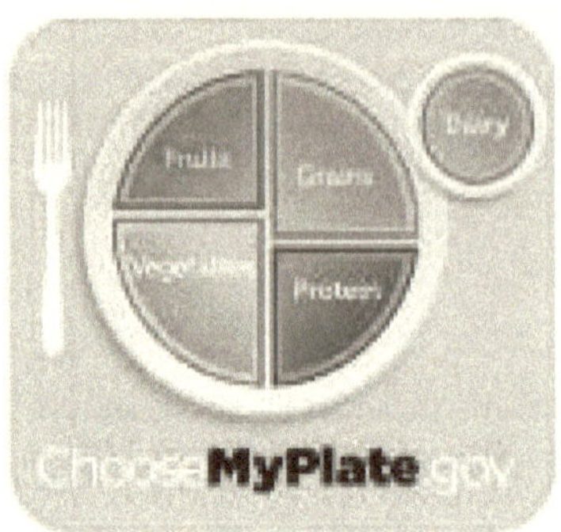

Source: U.S. Government, 2011. MyPlate.
http://blog.usa.gov/post/6148726974/myplate-replaces-food-pyramid

In 2010, the USDA acknowledged that the Food Pyramid diet had never been tested. It was designed to satisfy calorie needs, not nutrient requirements. Many nutritionists found that their patients were becoming obese, overweight, and sick despite following the USDA's carbohydrate-rich, grain-based diets.

These are the main problems with this diet:

> The excessive consumption of refined carbs or sugars

> a lack of high-quality nutrient rich natural oils or fats (such as butter, avocado, olive oil and coconut oil), which are essential for good health. There is actually no fat on the plate. In the food pyramid, healthy fats had been replaced by highly processed, unnatural vegetable oils like canola and soybean oil, margarines, and trans fats.
> pasteurized, homogenized fat-free milk

> Poorly prepared whole grains, pulses, and nuts that are high in antinutrients can harm absorption and deplete vital minerals

Patients felt healthier, had more energy, and lost weight when they started eating foods such as grass-fed butter. Their overall health improved. Learn more about the causes of obesity skyrocketing in this fascinating article: USDA's Pyramid Scheme.

Raw Food Diet

This diet is about eating food in its natural state, without any cooking. However, it allows for some foods to be processed at low temperatures to dry them. Although replacing junk food with organic raw foods is a significant step, it's not the final destination.

Raw foods are thought to contain more enzymes than cooked food. Cooking supposedly destroys many of these enzymes.

While this may be true up to a point. However, the real key to the answer is what your body can absorb. Many foods are more easily absorbed by cooking. The question is: Which food has the greatest net gain?

Today, most people eat cooked food. One exception is the practice of the aboriginal people who eat cooked meat after a kill in hunting. The liver, fat and kidneys are the best pieces to gain power and nutrients.

It is amazing that almost all primitive cultures cook most of their food. It is done to make food more digestible and to maximize nutrient absorption.

Andreas Moritz did an excellent job of critiquing the raw food diet in Timeless Secrets of Health and Rejuvenation. While he explained the reasons it works for a while, he also highlighted some of the real dangers of this type of eating over time. After cleansing the colon, raw foods can cause a weakening in the digestive system, bloating and deterioration to joints and arteries. This can lead to a decreased ability to absorb nutrients and an overall weakening condition. Moritz stated that all major ancient civilizations had traditionally prepared their food to avoid natural poisons found in raw foods.

Scientists now believe that the human brain's growth was due to the discovery of fire as a cooking method. This allowed for better nutrient absorption. This allowed for the brain to absorb more nutrients, which led to its significant increase in size.

"Heating our food unlocked nutrients: 100 percent is metabolized by our bodies, while raw foods only 30 to 40 percent." What makes us human? According to Study, Cooking is a Healthy Habit

"Meat and cooked food were necessary to provide the required calorie boost for a growing brain."

Moritz continued, "The initial surge in energy and vitality following a raw food diet does not result from vitamins. It is caused rather by the sudden mobilization and activation of the immune system that tries to counteract the massive amount of enzyme inhibitors, antibodies, and other nutrients found in [raw] foods."

Many anti-nutrients are found in plant foods to protect them against predators. Traditions taught that food must be properly cooked, soaked, or fermented in order to maintain their health. This is particularly important for beans, grains, and nuts.

For some, a detox diet that focuses on raw foods may be the best option. A raw food diet is not a good long-term option, except for those with strong constitutions. It might be better to mix it with cooked food. Raw foodists tend to be vegans. This has additional risks.

Raw foodists can also eat sprouted food. Although sprouting makes foods more digestible, it is not as effective as cooking the food. Raw food lovers may also enjoy sprouts, such as wheat grass and dried powdered varieties. These types of green foods can cause irritation. Powdered greens were supposed to be super-healthy, and I've had complete prostate/urinary shut downs!

This diet is best suited for certain climates. It is possible to become more sick if you eat raw food in northern climates.

It is important to eat food "in season". It is possible to eat mangos in Alaska in January, but it may not be the best food. You might be surprised to find out that fruits from faraway countries are not good.

Raw foods such as sauerkraut and fermented vegetables can be part of a healthy, well-balanced diet that maximizes enzymes. These foods are rich in enzymes that aid digestion and replenish the digestive fluids.

A fermentation process called lacto-fermentation improves the enzyme content of raw foods and, when combined with cooked food, compensates for any enzyme loss. It can also make food much easier to digest. The fermentation process produces lactic acid and good bacteria, which survive digestion and reach the intestines. Lacto-fermented foods are considered "super-raw."

Consuming too many raw foods when your body is not getting vitamin D from the sunlight will cause severe damage to your body. This is because raw foods, particularly tropical fruits, tell your body to stop releasing vitamin D.

Because of its high potassium content, the food itself is a sign that you are getting vitamin D from the sun.

If you are in the tropics, and outside in the sun, this would be fine. It doesn't work in all climates, if you don't get D from the sun. Your ileocecal valve, which is the connection between your large and small intestines, eventually fails to close completely and your entire digestive system suffers. Even the best quality food can be your enemy if it is not properly prepared or eaten in the wrong environment!

I believe that raw food should be eaten in moderation, ranging from 15% to 30% in the winter northerly zone. To find out if the raw food is healthy for you, I test it (see Chapter 10). While a raw food diet can be helpful for cleansing, it may not be the best option once you have completed that stage. You can return to cooking the majority of your food. Only in late summer or early fall can I eat fresh apples from my apple trees. Then I react to them. They are fine once they have been cooked in apple sauce.

We all need to eat more vegetables. For most vegetables, they should be cooked. Raw vegetable juices and salads can be eaten in moderation.

Avoid drinking fruit juices, unless you are able to enjoy them as a treat for a special occasion. You should eat fruit whole to get the full benefits of its fiber and bulk nutrients.

This doesn't necessarily mean that raw foods should be avoided. Raw food should not be a major part of your diet. Raw food can be great, but only in moderation according to the season and location.

The Vegetarian Diet

Many people consider the vegetarian diet superior. There are many variations of this diet. This diet has many flaws. It can be dangerous to eat the wrong type of dairy, i.e. pasteurized, and not raw. Vegetarians tend to eat too many sweets, phytic rich foods, nuts, and poorly prepared pulses. Vegetarians can become quite unhealthy. The life expectancy of people who eat more animal food in northern India is much higher than that of vegetarians.

Vitamin B12 is often lacking in vegetarians, as it isn't found in plant-based food. Vitamin B12: Vital Nutrient for Good Health provides more information.

To test for non-vegetarian food like eggs, fish and fowl, you can quickly test them to determine if they are positive. You may need to include them in your diet if they do. You should eat high-quality, grass-fed, organic meat products if you are looking for meat.

These articles will provide more information about the dangers associated with a vegetarian diet:

Twenty-Two Reasons Not to Go Vegetarian

Vegetarianism and Nutrient Deficiencies

The Vegetarian Myth by Lierre Keat

Lierre Keith outlined the dangers of eating a vegetarian diet, not only for our health but also for the environment.

She demonstrated clearly that mono-crop farming (never mind the animal-hungry factory farms) has depleted well above 90% of the U.S. topsoil, and is threatening the survival of many species.

Keith's book is a revelation and must-read for anyone who cares about the planet and their health. The subtitle of the book should read:

How our food choices and agricultural practices are threatening the planet and our health!

Hey, I was a vegan/vegetarian for many decades, and I ended up with a prostate problem. If you're a vegetarian, it might be worth considering the very near impossible: certain animal foods may be beneficial for both you and the earth!

Vegan Diet

It is basically a vegetarian diet, but it does not include animal products such as eggs or dairy. A large portion of this diet is raw. For information about vitamin and nutrient deficiency, please see the "Vegetarian Diet".

The China Study Diet

It is basically a vegetarian diet but does not include animal products such as eggs or dairy. This diet includes a lot of raw food. For information about vitamin and nutrient deficiencies, please see the following diets (raw or vegetarian).

China Study diet claims that vegetarian/vegan rural Chinese are healthier. Many of these conclusions are based on false assumptions or science. The China Study Myth provides a great insight and analysis into its claims.

Macrobiotic Diet

This is a variant of the vegan diet that allows for fish and plenty of vegetables, fruits, nuts, seeds, and vegetables. It's a diet high in complex carbohydrates, low in fat, and natural foods, with no dairy.

I discovered that many of these natural whole foods recommended by the FDA contain phytic acids. These anti-nutrients, also known as phytotates, can be so dangerous over time if they aren't removed by traditional methods such as fermenting and soaking. This is something I just discovered recently. I believe that phytic acids was the main factor in my prostate enlargement, even though I was eating a healthy diet!

For more information on phytic acids, see Chapter 3's section.

The macrobiotic diet gradually removes zinc (and other mineral) from the body. This is because the food preparation process is not done correctly. Zinc is an essential mineral for the prostate. I was a macrobiotic vegetarian for over 30 years and didn't know the dangers that it could lead to.

Alkaline Diet

This diet is also known as the pH diet or acid/alkaline diet. It is increasing in popularity. The body's alkaline or acid-forming status is what is used to classify food. This is a cleansing diet that I recommend, but not as a long-term nourishment diet.

This diet aims to maintain an alkaline body by eating foods that are alkaline. Acidic states are the root cause of many modern diseases and cancers. Many of the foods in my Food STOP List (see Chapter 6), as well as those I recommend for healthy eating, are too acidic.

They say that an ideal alkaline diet is one that is mostly vegetarian or vegan and sometimes raw with very little animal food. Because most of these foods are too acidic, it also reduces the consumption of bean and grain products.

The goal is to consume approximately 75% foods from the alkaline and 25% from the acidic lists. There will be many opinions from pundits about what constitutes acidity/alkalinity, but experts tend to agree on how the majority of foods are classified. The best chart is here: List Of Alkaline Foods.

For more information, go here:

Acid/Alkaline Diet

The Alkaline Diet

While this diet can be helpful for a brief time as a cleansing diet after a long-term poor diet with manufactured foods, it is not recommended long-term. While there are immediate benefits, the long-term effects of an alkaline diet can be detrimental.

While an alkaline diet can provide more nutrients than a junk diet for a time, it may prove costly in the long-term as you will not be able to absorb many of these nutrients, especially raw. Consuming most food in its raw form can cause health problems. (See the section on raw food diet).

The key to good health is what we absorb and how our bodies maintain these minerals.

The problem with this diet is that any food, even high-alkaline foods, can easily cause a negative reaction. This could be an acid-forming reaction due to the inflammatory response. This is what happened to me after I ate kale. It's a highly-recommended and alkaline vegetable. Some people can't eat that food.

This conclusion was drawn by Dr. Weston Price (a remarkable researcher who researched the diets and lifestyles of Native Americans, Gaelic, Eskimo and South Sea Islanders). He wrote that Dr. Price had compared the amounts of acid ash minerals and alkaline-ash minerals:

Acid ash foods dominated all diets except the South Sea. The important thing is that the total mineral content of every primitive diet was at minimum four times and sometimes more than tenfolds higher than that in modernized diets.

The Right Price by S. Fallon, www.westonaprice.org/basics/the-rightprice

You will notice the year of publication - 1935. Think about how much the modern diet will be deficient in minerals due to our depleting agrisoils!

I recommend that you only use the alkaline diet as a transition cleanse diet. You should also personally test every food (see Chapter 10 Personal Testing). Next, I will describe a nourishing diet.

Low Glycemic Diet/South Beach Diet

The glycemic index (GI) of food is what the proponents consider the best guide. Glycemic Index (GI), a numerical scale that indicates how quickly or high a food can raise blood sugar (blood glucose) levels, is what the Glycemic Index (GI). According to some, the lower the GI is, the healthier the food. Learn more at Wikipedia: Glycemic Index.

I think the entire concept of GI is flawed. It classifies whole grains such as rye bread as identical to jelly beans!

There is something wrong here!

Low glycemic foods are not good for you. Fats and cooking times have a negative impact on your glycemic index. Butter can be used on presoaked, cooked whole brown rice and whole grain sourdough bread to lower the glycemicindex. This means that the foods are absorbed slowly and not in one burst like high-GI foods.

It is not a scientific diet that counts, but properly prepared foods with high quality saturated oils. To find out if your body is ready for high-GI foods such as brown rice and whole grain sourdough bread, you can test it yourself. Make sure they are properly prepared and that you add good quality fats so they can be slowly absorbed.

Body Type Diets: Ayurvedic Diet/Blood Type Diet

Ayurvedic is a traditional and time-tested diet that is based on Ayurvedic principles of India. It identifies three main body types and shows which foods work best for each. Because it recognizes differences between body types, it has a lot to offer.

These are three books on this diet. The questionnaires will help you determine your body type.

The Timeless Secrets of Health and Rejuvenation

Ayurvedic healing, 2nd revised and expanded edition: A comprehensive guide

The Quantum Alternative to Growing Old: Ageless Body, Timeless Thought:

Ayurvedic recommendations are largely vegetarian. Please test your food to verify the suggestions. Otherwise, it might be too restrictive. It is difficult for me to follow this diet without experiencing reactions. This is especially true since many phytate foods are recommended by my diet. To minimize the effects of phytic acid, make sure to read Chapter 3's information on phytic acids reduction.

Ayurvedic diets often recommend too many tropical foods. We know this because we have seen it in raw form in hot climates. (See Chapter 3, Eat according to Your Climate).

This is a great starting point once you have identified your "type", but it's important to be cautious with the suggestions. You can take some of the ideas and then test the foods to see if they are compatible. There are many body types, and no one theory can explain them all. Ayurveda actually expands the basic 3-10 versions.

These same precautions apply to the blood type diet. The diet takes into account your blood type in order to determine what you should eat. It's scientifically based, just like the alkaline diet. However, it is important to test the water first and take it with a grain salt!

Many of the food suggestions I have been given by my blood type are not suitable for me. They either test negative or cause immediate reactions. Your uniqueness is the reality. Diet theories don't work long-term.

Learn more: Blood Type Diet by Dr. Lam.

Test foods for compatibility. You will discover what resonates with you and be amazed at the results. See Chapter 10. Your body's inner wisdom will know what it needs.

High-Carb-Low-Fat Diet or Low-Protein Diet; the Hunter-Gatherer Diet, Primitive Diet, or Paleo Diet; and the Low-Carb-High-Protein Diet

Because the questions of fat, proteins and carbohydrates are all common, I have grouped these diets together.

Weston Price, the researcher quoted above, said that a high-carb, low-fat diet was dangerous. Industrialized people, such as us, eat non-fermented carbohydrates. They avoid nutrient-dense food. Because these foods are all around, it is difficult for them to avoid highly processed and devitalized foods. These foods can lead to addiction and a diet that is dominated by additives!

Read CBC's article Food Cravings Engineered By Industry and Natural News's one: The Ultimate Craving - How Industry Designs Food to Be as Addictive As Narcotics (and Keeps us Coming Back For More).

Many people now believe that high-carb, low-fat diets are the main cause of obesity.

The dramatic rise in obesity over the past three decades is a result. It is deadly to consume too many sugary carb starches and sugar products made from white flour.

According to the Paleo diet, we should eat the same food our ancestors ate about 10,000 years ago before agriculture was invented. Paleo enthusiasts claim that the Paleo diet was high in protein and low in carbohydrates. Modern Paleo often suggests lean cuts of meat. It is a diet that is very different from the one our ancestors followed. The diet has too little fat and too many proteins, which can lead to toxicity and deficiencies.

Paleo diets should have adequate saturated fat. However, many Paleo dieters still struggle with carbs.

Enthusiasts believe that carbs weren't eaten back then, but roots and tubers were a staple of primitive diets. They were rich in digestible carbohydrates when prepared properly and were consumed with saturated natural fats.

The problem is similar to the low-carb-high-protein diets:

Protein powders are often added to diets to increase the protein content and reduce calories. This can lead to a diet that is unnaturally high-protein, something that primitive people avoided. Vitamin A is required for protein metabolism. A diet high in protein but low in fat can quickly deplete vitamin A stores. This can lead to serious consequences such as heart arrhythmias and kidney problems, autoimmune diseases, thyroid disorders, and even death. A negative calcium balance is also caused by a diet high in protein. This means that more calcium is lost than it is taken in. This can cause bone loss and nervous system disorders.

Adventures in Macro-Nutrient Land by S. Fallon and M. G. Enig, www.westonaprice.org/basics/adventures-in-macro-nutrient-land

You will see good results in the short-term with the high protein weight loss diet. Weight loss is possible. You will lose weight, but your body will eventually become toxic (ketosis), from the excessive intake of protein. This could lead to kidney disease, kidney stones, cancer, organ failure, kidney failure, high cholesterol, and osteoporosis!

These diets are superior to eating what most Americans eat (see Chapter 6). These diets may not be right for you. You can only find out if these diets are right for you by paying attention to their flaws and trying the food yourself (see Chapter 10).

Carbohydrates in whole grains and beans can be considered highly nutritious, provided they are prepared properly (soak, sprouted and leavened) as well as eaten with the highest quality saturated fats.

Another problem with these diets is the recommendation of low-fat or vegetable fats in place of saturated fats. Vegetable fats contain too many omega-6 fats. These fats can be extremely harmful if they are on the Food STOP List. We will discuss the dangers associated with low-fat diets in a later article. This article provides more information on low-fat diets: Low fat diets lead to cognitive decline and miss essential brain nutrients.

The Weston A. The Price Foundation's Health Topics is an extensive site of research that examines the best foods. It's well worth your time to read and search the site.

Remember, when researching online, it doesn't matter how much research you do or the insights you gain, the final test is to actually test the foods you are interested in before you eat them.

Mediterranean Diets

These diets, which are based on the Mediterranean culture's eating habits, have some positive points. However, many wrong conclusions have been made about fat and meat.

They advocate olive oil as an occasional oil, but not for primary use. They also deny the health benefits of high-quality saturated fats. Many recommend that you limit your intake of meats. It is a good idea to avoid toxic commercial meats, but it may be harmful to you if you exclude traditionally raised animals. It is also important to know the differences between pasteurized dairy products and raw milk dairy products.

You can read the discussion about these important issues in this book: fat, meat, and dairy.

Although it is great to use lots of vegetables, many of the grains used are not.

These diets are very refined and have all the nutrients removed. The pastas, breads, and other foods are no longer properly prepared as we have already discussed. See gluten-free diets below.

Weight Loss Diets

Many of these programs will sell you protein powders, shakes, and other concoctions. Be careful. Many of these products are manufactured with highly processed ingredients that contain GMO-derived corn, soy, and taste enhancers (neurotoxic substances). Many of these sweeteners are artificial or fructose. These sweeteners can be very toxic for your health.

There are more than 90 symptoms that aspartame toxicity can cause. These include anxiety attacks, brain cancers, breathing difficulties, depression, abdominal pain, dizziness and marked personality changes. Side effects of sucralone include dizziness and panic attacks, nausea, vomiting, diarrhea, swelling headaches, cramping, stomach pain, and dizziness.

The Weston A. has submitted a petition to the FDA for approval of aspartame. Price Foundation, www.westonaprice.org/2013-action-alerts/dairyindustry-petitions-fda-to-approve-aspartame Another article is: Aspartame Pathway.

Be aware of the so-called "diet" food and protein energy bars. Many contain artificial sweeteners such as Splenda and Equal. Both can cause neurodegenerative damage, gastrointestinal problems, and endocrine disruption.

Be aware of the chemical flavorings that are added to your food. These chemicals replace fat and other natural ingredients that have been removed in order to trick you.

A cleansing diet, such as raw juice, can be very effective for some people. As we know, cleansing is not for long-term as it can become problematic. Many dieters experience new symptoms or go back to their old ways after they stop eating properly.

Follow these diet suggestions if you are looking to lose weight. A nourishing, natural diet is the best way to lose weight permanently.

Gluten-free Diets

Many people can be severely affected by years of eating processed grains that are high in gluten, such as wheat, kamut and rye. According to the advocates of this diet, there is a way to completely avoid gluten.

This practice will be beneficial for you if you have a gluten allergy. Gluten-free foods can pose risks long-term. New conditions can develop if gluten-free grains such as rice are not prepared by soaking to lower the anti-nutrients (phytic Acid).

Many gluten-free products sold in supermarkets and health food stores today are filled with low quality ingredients such as vegetable fats, substitutes, sugars and GMOs. White rice is often used, but it is stripped of its nutrients, which can lead to weight gain.

Gluten intolerance is a common condition:

> The poor quality of modern commercial grains used in white bread, pastas, and other foods.

Because they are devoid of any vitamins, minerals, fiber, or other nutrients, they can be toxic to your body. This can cause health problems as the body is unable to properly digest or assimilate these foods. Refined white flour has been bleached with chlor and brominated using bromide. These poisonous chemicals have been linked with thyroid and organ damage.

Bread, and Why Avoid Most of It by Dr. Lawrence Wilson, drlwilson.com/ARTICLES/BREAD.htm

> The anti-nutrients (phytates in them) are especially bad for flaked and extruded puff cereals.

> Whole grains that have been prepared without any cooking, soaking, or fermentation

> The use of bran (very high levels in phytates), which can be very harmful to the

If you don't have the whole grain prepared properly for optimal digestion, gut is okay!

> The diet lacks high quality saturated fats such as butter from pastured cattles. This helps to digest the grains and minimizes any adverse reactions

You may actually find that you can gradually introduce whole grains with gluten into your diet if you get back to proper preparation!

It happened to me. After 35 years of eating grain without knowing how to prepare them safely and adding butter to aid digestion, I was forced to stop eating them. It lasted for one year. Gluten grains were the worst. Two years later, I am able to eat wheat, rye, and kamut provided I make them right! They are high in gluten. They contain a lot of gluten.

Conclusion

While many diets are popular, not all of them will work for everyone. Many of these diets have serious flaws which can worsen your overall health. You should take the advice of experts with a grain. Learn as much as you can and then test each food individually to determine if it is right for you (see Chapter 10).

The next chapter of the STOP lists will cover things you should absolutely avoid.

Chapter 6: The "STOP" Lists

This section explains what you should stop eating. Food can be a medicine or a poison. We have the power to choose not to fall prey to our bad habits.

Many of the toxic foods we consume are addictive and toxic. Because not all toxins can be eliminated through the overburdened elimination system, some toxins can be forced into the body's outer tissues. One result is weight gain.

Our digestion suffers when our gut becomes a toxic wasteland. Chronic health conditions can develop. Our prostates bear a huge burden. To give your body the best chance of natural healing, it is important to eliminate toxic foods.

Sensitivities and Allergies

Chronic conditions are those that affect most people every day, rather than an acute disease or infection. Chronic conditions are closely linked to allergies and sensitivities. Practitioners in natural health know that many patients with chronic or long-term conditions have one or more allergies.

What is an allergy? Allergies are when the body's immune systems produces antibodies in response to repeated exposure to an antigen or substance that is normally harmless.

Disruptive and unpleasant symptoms will most likely be felt in the area where the defense reaction is more obvious. If the reaction occurs in the nose, sinuses, or lungs, extreme mucus congestion can occur and breathing problems may result.

An allergic reaction in the prostate can lead to an enlarged prostate or cancer. Ovarian cysts may be caused by a similar immune reaction in women.

Constipation can lead to toxic absorption through the thin rectal wall. Toxins are carried right through the prostate every time you pee. It matters what you eat!

The Gut

As I learn more about healing, I am more aware of how important our digestive system is for our health and the progress that we make.

Many people have compromised digestive systems. This is due to decades of abuse of antibiotics, inoculations and pesticides.

These symptoms are often a sign of a compromised digestion, also known as leaky gut:

> constipation and bloated stomach

> Diarrhea or irregular bowels

> Sore and/or coated tongue

> Frequent gas and cramping

> awful-smelling bowel movements

> stomach aches and hemorhoids

> Bad breath or heartburn

These symptoms are a sign that your colon and intestinal tract aren't working optimally.

Your bowels can become contaminated with dangerous toxins. This can lead to food sensitivities, allergies, and other serious health issues.

Antibiotics destroy both the good and the bad flora in your intestines. This can lead to a compromised digestion. Overeating is prevented by your gut flora. Overeating can be caused by antibiotics!

The body's digestive system can be severely damaged by antibiotics. Sometimes antibiotics are necessary and can help us avoid serious health problems. In 90% of cases, however, antibiotics are unnecessary and prescribed too often for minor conditions. Side effects are a part of every drug.

The moral of the story is that almost everyone has a compromised digestion tract. The consequences are allergies, sensitivities and chronic health issues, as well as a tired body that takes pleasure out of living.

You can make progress in healing by changing your diet and improving your health.

It is not a straight line up! It can be difficult because of how our digestive system has been abused.

You can do everything you can to increase the friendly bacteria in your gut and make it more efficient at destroying the undesirable critters. This can be done by optimizing your diet and testing for sensitive foods. You can also take probiotics such as digestive enzymes, acidophilus, glutamine, and FOS.

Candida yeast syndrome is characterized by sugars of all types, with the most severe being fructose. Stop them!

Our gut is the centre of our immune system. All fermented foods, including natural raw milk yogurt, kefir, sauerkraut and kimchi, must contain friendly bacteria. These probiotics and friendly bacteria will help your digestion and support your healing journey. If you are positive, please start small (1/2 teaspoon) Next, increase slowly.

Your tongue is your best indicator of how you're doing. If your tongue isn't pink and uncoated, you know that you need to work!

Take a look at the following list to see if you can make sense of it.

The Food STOP List

You should follow my Food STOP List as closely as possible as these foods have become so toxic, de-nourished and altered that they are almost foreign to our bodies.

You can learn how to test food items to determine if they're good or not. These "Non-Food" products should be stopped for prostate health:

> Stop eating processed food. Cookies, candies and muffins are all examples. Avoid most things you see in supermarkets today.

> Stop eating most commercial, conventionally-grown, depleted, pesticide-contaminated fruits and vegetables.

> Reduce the use of refined sweeteners like fructose and sugar, dextrose, glucose, fructose corn syrup (recently found mercury in more than 40% of products tested). Bottled fruit juices, energy drinks, etc.

> Stop using artificial sweeteners and sugar substitutes like Splenda and Aspartame brands.

Stop eating hydrogenated, partially hydrogenated fats, trans oils and oil. Canola oil (the GMO first food made from toxic Rapeseed Oil), corn oil, soybean oil, margarine and Becel, as well as cottonseed oil and safflower or safflower oils. You can replace it with organic butter, ghee and lard. Find out more at Know Your Fats. Canola oil is another victory of food technology over common sense. This article explains the dangers of soybean oil.

> Avoid consuming pasteurized or homogenized milk products and other dairy products. You can replace them with raw milk products (ideal), or small quantities of organic ones (nowhere as beneficial as raw). Visit A Campaign for Real Milk to learn more.

> Avoid eating factory-farmed eggs, fowl and all types of processed meats. It is best to replace with organic, grass-fed, and free-range products.

Stop using salt from commercial sources. Instead, use sea salt.

Health food store products may contain some of the restrictions mentioned above. Many foods found in health food stores are unhealthy.

> Do not consume Genetically Modified Foods (GMO)

Irradiated and Engineered foods. American Academy of Environmental Medicine issued this warning: Genetically Modified Foods.

Avoid eating salmon and other fish from commercial farms unless they are organic. These fish are fed antibiotics and toxic feeds.

Avoid mercury-rich fish such as swordfish, king mackerel and tilefish. These wild fish should be eaten instead of farmed: catfish, flounder and haddock (Atlantic), herring (North Atlantic), mackerel, tilefish, grouper, marlin, orange roughy, walleye, tuna, salmon, sole (Pacific), scallop, shrimp, sole, squid, tilapia, freshwater trout, whitefish.

This consumer guide contains a comprehensive list of the best and most harmful fish: The Consumer Guide to Mercury In Fish.

Avoid canned foods. The can linings are toxic (coated in BPA) and the food is devitalized.

- Stop drinking caffeinated drinks and commercial products.
- Stop using powdered protein concoctions or mixes.

Stop eating processed cereals, grains and nuts, as well as granolas. They are high in phytic acid (phytates), and can deplete the body's vital minerals. To reduce the irritation, these foods must be soaked in water first, which can include organic grains, seeds, and nuts. Extruded foods, such as flakes and puffed cereals (often coated in oils and sugars), rice cakes and shredded cereals are the worst.

Consume no soy products such as soymilk, soy cheese, and frozen soy desserts. They contain high levels of phytotic acid. They can also be harmful, particularly in relation to hormones. You can eat tempeh, miso, and tamari made from fermented soybeans. Avoid non-organic brands. They are often sprayed with herbicides, pesticides, and may also contain GMO soybeans. Only use organic brands. For more information, see this article called "Soy Alert" and this article entitled "The Truth About Unfermented Soy and Its Harmful Side Effects".

Fluoridated water should be stopped. Fluoridation causes hypothyroidism, immune deficiency, weight gain, and heart disease. This article Fluoridation: A Scam of the Century, and this article Fluoride Depletes Iodine In the Body, Causing Hypothyroidism & Immune Deficiency.

Avoid drinking chlorinated water from cities. The highly toxic chemical chlorine can easily mix with other trace contaminants to create highly carcinogenic chemicals. Get rid of chlorine and other toxic substances from your water.

Avoid grilling meats on flames that cause cancer by burning fats. Instead, slow cook your meat.

Stop eating commercial foods that contain monosodium glutamate (MSG), and other food enhancers such as vegetable protein, hydrolyzed proteins, hydrolyzed plant proteins, plant protein extracts, sodium caseinates, calcium caseinates, yeast extracts, textured protein and hydrolyzed oatmeal flour.

Stop eating at fast food restaurants that serve large quantities of Food STOP List products.

• Stop using nonstick and aluminum cookware. Instead, use stainless steel, cast iron or stoneware, as well as glass and ceramic pots, pans, and plates.

> Quit smoking and quit drinking distilled alcohol. Red wine and small-batch organic beers can be consumed in moderation.

> Avoid as many prescriptions as possible, and instead choose natural medicines that can be used for very short periods.

> Stop getting vaccines. This article explains the dangers of vaccines as well as the effects on your immune system.

Disposable coffee cups and take-out containers should be thrown out. These cups contain both formaldehyde preservatives and styrene (another additive). Both have been added to the federal government's 12th Report on Carcinogens.

• Stop using the microwave. It can cause food to be ruined.

The Food STOP List lists the modern killer foods that are the main cause of today's epidemic levels of chronic diseases and problems with the prostate. We are highly toxic to cannibals, overfed and undernourished!

Good news! When you replace unhealthy foods with whole, real food, you can regain your health and taste the delicious, real foods. You can grow your own food and enjoy fresh, delicious food.

Stop Eating Farmed Fish

Farm-raised fish can be dangerous for your health in many ways. All animals require the same optimal diet for good health.

Fish were designed to eat plankton and insects, other fish, plankton and other aquatic creatures, but not corn, grains or pork. This is an unnatural diet. All species of fish are fed vitamins and antibiotics. Fish meat can also be dyed. Their flesh may not have the same natural colors as wild fish due to the unnatural diet. Synthetic pigments are also used in their diet.

You are also eating PCBs, dioxins and toxaphene if you eat farmed seafood. These chemicals don't sound good for your health! These are not foods! Studies have consistently shown that mercury levels in farmed fish are higher than those in wild fish.

Stop Eating Microwaved Food

Russian scientists did extensive research into microwaves. Microwave cooking can destroy the vitamins B, C, and E that are associated with heart disease prevention and cancer prevention. Microwaving can also cause the loss of trace minerals in your food. Microwave cooking is nutritionally ineffective. People who eat microwave meals have higher rates of cancer cell growth.

He wrote the following:

William P. Kopp, Reporting for AREC Research's Forensic Research Document, now states that "the effects of microwaved foods byproducts are permanent and long-lasting within the human body. All microwaved foods are altered in such a way that minerals, vitamins, and nutrients are reduced or eliminated. Or, the body absorbs compounds that cannot be broken up. . ."

A classic experiment was conducted in which 2,000 cats were fed only water and food that had been previously heated in the microwave oven. The most nutritious and natural foods were chosen. All the cats died within six weeks. The surprising test result revealed that the cats were not well-fed and their cells had virtually no nutrient-components. Despite all their nutritious food, the cats died from starvation. The microwave turned their food into poisonous poison.

A. Moritz shares timeless secrets of health and rejuvenation

Click this link to learn more about the dangers of microwave ovens: Ninety percent of homes contain this health risk.

Click this link to learn more about the dangers of microwave cooking.

Imagine what microwaved food does to your prostate and you!

Personal Care Items STOP List

Your skin is the largest organ in your body and absorbs everything you put on it. Many body care products contain toxic chemicals that are easily absorbed by your skin.

Your liver and kidneys will then have to deal with these chemicals. Over time, these toxic chemicals can affect your prostate.

Cosmetics and body products that are labeled as "natural" can be suspect, since they don't conform to any code or standard. Marketing uses the word "natural" too often and in misleading ways.

You can only find out if a product's safety by searching the SIRI MSDS Index. This index will contain specific ingredients:

> cocoamide DEA and diethanolamine, Triethanolamine, TEA, Triethanolamine, and MEA

> mercury

> parabens

> propylene glycol, propylene oxide, polyethylene glycol

> Petrolatum and Coal Tar

> phthalates

> sodium lauryl sulfate, sodium laureth sulfate

> sodium fluoride

Your toxic load is not increased by using toothpaste, shaving cream, shampoos, conditioners, shampoos, and aftershaves. Products without ingredients should be read.

The Environmental Working Group maintains a huge database of body care products, including shampoos, cosmetics, and sunscreens. All are rated according to their toxicity. EWG's Skin Deep cosmetics Database makes it easy to find safe products and evaluate the ones you use.

EWG's Sunscreen guide and Not So Sexy report about hidden chemicals in perfumes and colognes are also available.

Avoid using traditional body care products to prevent prostate problems. Be smart! Be aware of what you're using.

Safe products may be more expensive, but they are better for your health. This saves you a lot of money over the long-term and prevents unnecessary suffering. This article gives you a great view of the subject: How to heal yourself in 15 days by cleaning up your skin exposure.

You can find great sources for body care products made by small-scale producers at the Organic Consumer Association website, or here at Amazon: Organic Body Care Products on Amazon.

I recommend that organic body care products be purchased from trusted manufacturers and that the product passes your personal testing. You can be sure that your products are safe by testing them every now and again to make sure there are no adverse reactions.

One of my favourite brands that goes a long distance for the dollar is Dr. Bronner's extremely high quality and pure line soaps and shampoos: Dr. Bronner's Body Care. Try the almond scent. It is my favorite.

These are some of my favorite body care tips:

> Start the day by taking a teaspoon of coconut oil or organic sesame oil and swirling it around in your mouth for 5-15 minutes. This helps to absorb any toxins that have been released over the night. It is highly effective.

> Use a tongue scraper after brushing to get rid of even more toxins your tongue.

> Body oiling: oil your body every now and again, especially if it is dry or has been exposed to the sun. Apply a few drops of organic coconut oil, sesame oil or olive oils to your entire body. Olive oil is my favorite. After waiting a while, you can then take a shower. Only use soap or shampoo on the underarms, crotch and hair.

Household Products STOP List

The dangers of household products, including laundry detergents and dish liquids, as well as floor cleaners and air cleaners, are the same. Both "natural" and conventional versions can be toxic. You may think that water is enough to wash it away. The vapors seep into your skin and get into your air. The traces remain in your clothing and penetrate your skin.

The first step in regaining your health is to stop the toxic assault. Keep in mind how close your prostate is to your bladder and rectum. Because of its proximity to these organs, your prostate can absorb toxins easily.

Don't believe me? Learn for yourself. This article outlines the chemical compounds found in different rooms and products within your home. Toxic Household Chemicals is a short overview. Then, test them yourself to make sure they are safe.

These are toxic household products that need to be stopped.

• Stop using fabric softeners and commercial laundry products. Use organic products that contain safe ingredients instead.

> Stop using deadly mothballs. They are toxic and have been banned in Europe. Instead, use natural alternatives such as sandalwood, citronella and cloves camphor/eugenin. For more information, see this article: Get Rid Of Moth Balls And Other Harmful Insecticides. Use Natural Alternatives.

> Avoid all commercial household cleaners and cleaners. Here are some safe and affordable alternatives: Natural Products and Household Cleaners.

Use plastic containers for food storage that have the numbers 3, 6, and 7 on the bottom of the recycling codes. BPA is a chemical that mimics estrogen and can be very dangerous to the prostate. Code #7 plastics often contain BPA. Hot food can be absorbed more easily if it is placed in plastic containers. Instead, use glass storage containers.

> Get rid of commercial air fresheners, perfumed candles and other fragrances. Use essential oil diffusers or beeswax candles instead.

The FDA has not approved any of these synthetic chemicals in household products as safe for human consumption. Anything that comes in contact with your body should be avoided. All body care products should be replaced with organic products that contain safe ingredients.

Although you may believe this is a long list, the truth is that we have so severely compromised our health, it is now time to return to trusted, safe products. Give your body a break! Stop "death by a thousand cuts!"!

Vista Magazine issue #75 features an article about chemicals:

The FDA has registered over 80,000 chemicals for industrial use.

US Environmental Protection Agency. Only 250 of these tests can be performed medically. To assess the level of contamination in the average person, the health agencies have taken samples from people. The health agencies tested for 210 chemicals and found that 167 were present in the individuals tested. There were 91 chemicals found in an average person.

It is obvious that all of us are toxic in some way or another. It's not surprising that we are losing the war against cancer, Alzheimer's, diabetes, thyroid disease and other chronic degenerative diseases.

The Obesity-Toxicity Connection by S. Kuprowsky, issuu.com/beaudrystudio/docs/vista_issue75

Start to clean out your entire house. All of these toxic products should be replaced with healthy and organic products. It's not easy to make changes and stop doing things if you want your health to improve, but it is worth it!

Orange TKO is my favorite super-concentrated organic household cleanser. It can be used in spray bottles.

Orange TKO is a citrus cleaner/degreaser that is made from the orange peel. It's an emulsifier that doesn't contain synthetic chemicals, petroleum distillates or detergents. It is 100% non-toxic, biodegradable, environmentally friendly and biodegradable. Orange TKO is a concentrated form of the product. It can be dilute with water to tackle the most difficult industrial cleaning problems. However, it can also be used safely in the home around children and pets. Orange TKO is safe for use in the home for all cleaning needs.

Orange TKO is a non-profit organization dedicated to the preservation of the environment

Here are two quick tips to help you use this incredible cleaner. Always shake the spray bottle before using it. Let it sit for between 10 and 30 seconds before wiping. TKO works like a charm and is very affordable! You can now get rid of all commercial toxic material.

This article contains more information about the dangers associated with common household materials.

Yikes! It's no wonder that prostate disease is so common in the West!

Pest Problems?

Organic Pest Control is a safe and effective household product that can replace toxic chemicals. These products are made from safe, organic ingredients that work better than toxic chemicals to your garden and lawn. These products are great for eliminating pests such as wasps and ants from your home.

This is an easy way to get rid of many ants. You will need a small cover to dissolve the borax powder and sugar into water. You will need about 1/2 teaspoon of borax and 1 teaspoon+ sugar. It attracts ants, so they eat it. Then they return it to their nest to die. They will be gone in a few days.

Get rid of all the junk in your home. Get rid of all the junk! Organic household products are a great way to fill your home.

You should not ignore the importance of household products for your health. There are no shortcuts to a healthy prostate. Only use safe products in your home.

Using Safe Cookware

Are you looking for the best cookware?

Glass and ceramic beakers can be used in a laboratory where it is important that the containers do not contaminate the experiment. Ceramic and glass are non-reactive or inert. . .

My goal is not to scare, but to help you understand why disease can arise based on what we do. Knowledge is power. Start by learning how to make changes, and then gradually substituting healthier options. They will eventually add up, and your health will improve.

Consider the reactivity and use non-reactive cookware whenever you can.

R. Wood offers healthy cookware

www.rebeccawood.com/health/healthy-cookware/

This article further demonstrates the dangers associated with nonstick cookware:

Be Informed: Non-Stick Pans Pose Danger

Below is a list with links to safe cookware:

> Natural Stoneware Bakeware

> Ceramic Cookware

> Glass Cookware

> Cast Iron Cookware

> Stainless Steel Cookware

Conclusion

Yes, it is difficult to break old habits. All I can do for you is to encourage. If you are looking for great health, the road ahead is easy. You may not want to go on the same road that you've been on. The most important journey of your life is up to you!

What I propose is that you return to foods from 100 years ago, before they were contaminated by food processing and other agricultural practices that created a toxic time bomb. I will go into more detail in Chapter 7 about these healthy foods.

Chapter 7: The Whole Wide World of Food and What You Should Eat

It is a daunting task to reconcile all the contradicting information available from many health sources and well-meaning professionals. Food is unique to each person, due to our individual preferences and dislikes. It is not an easy task to decide what food you should eat!

My approach is different than others. First, eliminate all known harmful foods. Then analyze the data to determine which foods are best for you. Next, find out what works best for you. This is the last step on your journey to good health.

Let's try to agree on some principles.

> Food is powerful medicine. It can heal or cause harm. The quality of our food has an impact on our health because it is the daily input that sustains our cells.

Our food can either help or hurt us. Harmful effects may not be immediately apparent or take a while to notice. While some people may not feel the effects of toxic, nutrient-poor food for many years, others can be sensitive to food that is unsafe and can suffer from them for decades or even decades. The severity of the disease can become severe when it finally surfaces, sometimes decades later.

> Because we are all unique and individual, every diet should be tailored to each person. You may find something that is good for me to be detrimental. It doesn't matter what the popularity or research is about a food, herb, or supplement. We are the masters and must discover for ourselves what works. This means that we need to start

with general guidelines and then do our own testing to confirm their effectiveness.

> All things change, even our bodies. They are constantly changing and need different inputs every day. You may find a food that isn't good for you today, but it might be great tomorrow or next year.

> More than just food, what we eat includes other inputs such as liquids like water and substances that pass through our skin.

Real Food List

People who eat real food every day are healthier and more likely to live long. The evidence is evident in the isolated communities found today in remote areas and mountains that practice these time-proven practices:

> Choose grass-fed, free-roaming, pastured meats. Also, eat fowl free to roam and feed on scraps or insects.

> Consume eggs from free-range birds and feed on insects and scraps; these eggs are rich and healthy and will have deep yellow yolks.

> Consume vegetables and fruits that have been grown in healthy soils without any pesticides or toxins.

> Consume healthy fats and oils.

> Consume grains, beans, pulses, nuts, and seeds that have been prepared using the traditional method of souring, fermenting, and soaking before cooking.

> Enjoy wild foods in their season (e.g., mushrooms, berries, nettles, etc.
).

> Consume real sea salt, and sea vegetables rich in trace elements and minerals.

> Only use natural sweeteners that are minimally processed from plants, bees, and trees.

> Make tea from herbs and spices grown at home or locally.

> Consume clean, uncontaminated water.

> Inhale clean, unpolluted oxygen-rich air.

> Increase your exposure of natural sunlight.

This food guide isn't bad, except that it doesn't explain the differences between grass-fed milk, fats, and meat. Don't ignore the soy recommendations. Honest Food Guide.

Your medicine is food. Supplements cannot replace the complex structure of nutrients real food provides. Real food is the basis of your health.

Fats

Fats are the most important food due to their ability to heal or harm us, and because they have the highest calories of all food groups. Yet fats are complex because there are so many perspectives.

Even mainstream medical organizations, not just holistic sites, now say that people need to reduce their intake of saturated fats in order to improve their prostate health. Many people believe that all fats are bad and should be cut. . . The low-fat diet crusaders.

It is true that saturated fats today are toxic. Numerous toxins, hormones, and antibiotics are concentrated in the fatty tissue of factory-farmed animals as well as in dairy fats. These toxic foods increase the risk of developing prostate cancer and other diseases. The countries with the highest levels of prostate disease are those that consume the most animal fats and animal foods.

Could it be possible that the fats we eat and the toxins they contain are more dangerous than the fat we eat? This is my opinion, and it's something that health experts often overlook.

Our animal fat must come from grass-fed, healthy fowl and not from poisoned animals.

Traditional cultures revered fat (mostly saturated fats), as well as the benefits it had for health. Saturated fats include animal fat, butter, and coconut oil. If they had to hunt only one animal in winter, they would have to survive on a diet that contained very little fat. They often died from a low-fat, protein-rich rabbit diet.

This article explains the dangers of low fat diets.

This major study is worth mentioning: The American Journal of Clinical Nutrition published a report in October 2010 stating that saturated fats were not associated with increased risk of heart disease (CHD), stroke, or cardiovascular disease (CVD)!

Conclusions: A meta-analysis prospective epidemiologic studies

It was found that there is not enough evidence to conclude that dietary saturated fat is linked with an increased risk for CHD [coronary hearts disease] or CVD [cardiovascular diseases].

P. W. Siri Tarino, Q. Meta-analysis of prospective cohort studies evaluating the association of saturated fat with cardiovascular disease Sun, F. B. Hu and R. M. Krauss

[ajcn.nutrition.org/content/early/2010/01/13/ajcn.2009.27725.abstrac %20](ajcn.nutrition.org/content/early/2010/01/13/ajcn.2009.27725.abstrac%20)

This proves that saturated fats are not dangerous. This study's findings should be taken a step further. I believe the rise in heart disease and other chronic conditions such as prostate disease, in modern society can be attributed to:

> The highly processed, harmful vegetable oils that are being promoted by almost all government agencies and organizations, such as the American Cancer Society or the American Heart Association. These fats are not good for the heart and brain.

> The altered nature of commercial saturated oils from modern agribiz techniques with all its toxins, and omega fat imbalances.

Good Fats to Eat

My prostate continued to suffer despite my diligent following of the recommendations of natural health experts and pundits. I had tried to reduce my fat intake and eliminate saturated fat. I was following the advice of eminent practitioners who were well-researched, published and successful.

I conclude that the recommendations of these doctors are incorrect because they only consider the statistics. For example, the statement "greater fat equals greater prostate disease" may seem true, but the research shows it to be false. These practitioners draw incorrect conclusions from data, much like urologists who believe that aging is the cause of prostate disease.

The problem is not high-quality, grass-fed saturated oils, but saturated fats from poisonous animals and modern vegetable fats containing excessive omega-6s or toxins. Toxins and imbalances in omega-6s and toxins are the problem!

Recent scientific research has shown that healthy saturated fats, such as those found in pasture-raised, grassfed animal meat and butter, and from coconut oil and natural sources like wild salmon are essential for healthy brain and heart health, and cancer prevention.

According to the Weston A. According to the Price Foundation, animal fats are rich in nutrients that can protect against heart disease and cancer. Consumption of large quantities of vegetable oils is associated with higher rates of heart disease and cancer.

Read Protect Yourself From Prostate Cancer by Simply Changing Your Diet.

Saturated fats rich in nutrients such as butter from free-grazing cattle and coconut oil are good choices. Choose natural meat fats over lean cuts when you eat high-quality meat. This is contrary to all the propaganda!

These are the foods that sustained our ancestors through the ages.

Are you concerned about your cholesterol? This book will help you dispel many myths about cholesterol.

This article exposes the myths surrounding cholesterol from saturated fat as the main harbinger for heart disease and death.

Quality saturated fat is the best choice you can make in regards to fat. It is easy to test if my advice is right for your body (see Chapter 10). You will be surprised at how well your body responds high quality saturated fats!

You will be surprised at the results of testing the commercial fats (soy and corn, safflower, and the margarines).

Ghee, also known as clarified butter, is a wonderful source for the highest quality saturated fats from grass-fed cows. Ghee is stable and delicious without refrigeration, with a long shelf-life. It is packed in jars and shipped unrefrigerated. Ghee is an excellent source of the highest quality saturated fats and it is lactose-free. Ghee can be used plainly or as a cooking ingredient because it has a high smoking point. For more information, visit the Pure Indian Foods website.

Omegas

The ratio of omega-6 to Omega-3 is another thing to think about. We are lacking in omega-3s. We are now eating too many omega-6s, which has led to a drastic change in the ratio of omega-6 to Omega-3 fats.

This is evident in certain aspects of our diet, such as meats bought at a regular grocery store or restaurant. For example, grass-fed beef has omega-6 and omega-3 fatty acid ratios that are close to the healthy 2:1. Grain-fattened commercial beef is what most people eat. It contains fat in an unbalanced ratio, ranging from 20:1, 30 and 50 to omega-6!

The anti-tumor effects of omega-6 polyunsaturated fat acids (from soybean, corn, safflower, and other vegetable oils), outweigh the protective effects of omega-3s.

Jon Barron's article Fats and Oils Made Simple is available.

Avoid These Bad Fats

Stop the soy, corn, safflower, sunflower, canola, hydrogenated and partially-hydrogenated oils and margarines completely, even the health food store or organic varieties. Don't believe the hype about how healthy these oils are. Another excellent article about fat is The Great Con-ola.

Olive, coconut, and avocado oils should be used in moderation. Extra virgin oils of these oils should always be used. Experimenter-expressed sesame and peanut oils, as well as flax, almond, walnut, and flax oils, are acceptable. However, I do not recommend that you use these oils for daily or occasional use. Avoid refined oils. Trans fats can be dangerous and highly processed.

Margarine

Let's look at the process of making margarine. The heat is so high that vegetable oils can be melted. The oils turn rancid when they are heated to extreme high temperatures. To ensure solidification, a nickel catalyst is added to the heated oils. This is where deodorants and colorants can be added.

The final solidification process produces harmful trans-fatty acid, which can be fatal.

They are extremely carcinogenic. Margarine also contains harmful ingredients like emulsifiers and preservatives. They can cause cancer. Hexane is not something to be consumed by itself, since it is made from crude oil. Sterols, which are estrogen compounds, can cause endocrine issues and may also contribute to sexual inversion. Most margarine products use BHT (Butylated Hydroxytoluene). This ingredient can also cause side effects like dizziness, abdominal pain, nausea, and vomiting.

*Why Organic, Raw Butter will Benefit Your Health by S. Botes,
www.naturalnews.com/031497_raw_butter_health.html*

Eat More Fats!

Increase your intake of good fats! Yes, I did say increase them. These were the most prized foods of our forefathers. The rich fatty nutrients found in the animal's fat and organs were prized by these people. The internal organs of an animal were often consumed immediately after a hunt. Dogs were only allowed to eat the lean cuts if they had no other food. Our ancestors knew exactly what they needed to thrive and survive.

Pre-agricultural people were larger and more muscular than those who had been exposed to agriculture. They also had fewer cavities. As the population grew through agriculture, the amount of good fat in their diets decreased and they had less access to high-quality nutrition.

Our ancestors were able to preserve their food from the harmful effects of phytic acid once they learned how to soak and ferment grains. Due to poverty, wars, and a lack access to animals, too many reliance on grains that lack good saturated fats led to a decline of health. You can see this in the skeletons as well as dental records.

You can read more in this book: An Edible History Of Humanity by Tom Standage.

The health of hunter-gatherers is actually better than that of the earliest farmers. . . The farm produces a more varied and balanced diet than hunting or gathering. . . Cereal grains are good for calories but do not provide all the essential nutrients. . .

A high-carb diet combined with poor quality saturated fats can lead to serious health problems.

We were also led down a wrong path by false assumptions and corporate profit. Modern oils are very profitable for the industry.

Modern oils have replaced healthy fats, and factory-farmed animals have replaced them with toxic, factory-farmed ones. This has led to a decline in prostate health and an increase in cardiovascular disease. The Weston A. The Weston A:

Saturated fats, with a healthy omega 6 to 3 ratio, suppress inflammation. This is an important benefit in reducing benign prostate hyperplasia (BPH), enlargement of prostate and other forms of prostate cancer that are becoming more common in modern times.

Summary on Good Fats

Saturated Fats

> The majority of saturated fats are found in animal fats (from pastured livestock) in meat, butter, ghee, and tropical oils (e.g. coconut oil and palm kernel oil).

Daily recommended intake of saturated fat: 2 to 4 tablespoons.

Monounsaturated Fats

> Cod liver oil. Monounsaturated fats are the predominant constituents.

> Daily monounsaturated fat recommendation: 1 to 2 tablespoons (or small handfuls of nuts).

Safe Polyunsaturated Fats

> Most of the polyunsaturated fats found in flax oil, walnut oil (evening primrose oil), black currant oil, and borage oil are from flax oil.

> Daily intake of polyunsaturated fats: 1-2 teaspoons.

For more information, read this article called "The Skinny on Fats". Always choose extra virgin oils.

The unsafe polyunsaturated oils that are used in modern vegetable oils are the most dangerous. While the above oils are acceptable, the soybean,

grape, cottonseed, sunflower, canola and safflower polyunsaturated oils that are not safe are not good oils. To be made, they require extreme high heat and pressure as well as chemical solvent processing. This makes them toxic. These oils can be deadly. Chronic disease has increased significantly since their introduction. These oils should be avoided even if they are organic. Use them sparingly at best.

You can read more about PUFA here: What is it? And Why Should It Be Avoided?

Your hormones will be regulated by healthy fats such as those found in avocados, pastured eggs and full-fat raw dairy milk, cheese, yogurt, butter, ghee and grass-fed meats and their fats, wild salmon and coconut oil. A diet rich in healthy fats can help keep your testosterone levels high and prevent prostate cancer. You will feel fuller and can even lose weight. Your libido will also increase as a side effect. This is a problem!

Oil and Fat Smoke Points

Oil can smoke if it is used in cooking. Oil that has started smoking can cause it to turn into a carcinogen, which can lead to cancer. This is why barbecued meats that catch fire from the oil are dangerous.

Below are the oil smoke points for recommended oils, sorted by temperature. The oils listed in bold font represent safe oils that can be used daily. You may also use other oils occasionally. Oils not listed below are considered unsafe and should not be used at any temperature (e.g. canola oil).

Temperature	Oil
225°F	Flaxseed Oil, Unrefined – *do not heat this oil!*

320°F	Peanut Oil, Unrefined; Walnut Oil, Unrefined
350°F	**Butter**; **Coconut Oil**; Sesame Oil, Unrefined
361–390°F	**Lard**; Olive Oil; Extra Virgin Macadamia Nut Oil
410°F	Sesame Oil
430°F	Almond Oil; Hazelnut Oil
482°F	Ghee
491°F	Avocado Oil, Unrefined

Protein

Another controversial topic is protein. High protein is a topic that has been controversial. It is the quality fat that we need, but are told by the punditry not to use. Even worse, we are instructed to use toxic commercial vegetable oils!

Your cravings for protein will decrease if you consume enough natural saturated fats. Your metabolism will be greatly affected by nutrient-rich broths that include animal fats, butter, and coconut oils.

Personal testing is the best way to determine how much protein you need. Keep in mind the portion size rule (section called Meat), or better yet, test your body personally to determine the best amount of protein (see Chapter 10, Personal Testing).

Vegetarians should ensure that all dairy products are from grass-fed animals. Whole grains and beans are great sources of high-quality protein. To remove harmful phytates from grains, beans, pulses and nuts, soak or ferment your grains before sprouting or boiling.

Read Grass-fed Basics for more information on protein. You can also find grass-fed milk and meat on this website.

Poultry and Eggs

Avoid commercial products that contain poor feed, confinement, or manufacturing additives. These products can be especially dangerous to your prostate.

The omega-6 fats in commercial eggs are more than those found in organic, free-range eggs, which have higher levels of the beneficial omega-3 fats.

According to some health experts, eggs are the worst food you can eat. Others say the exact opposite. Natural News article: Eggs--Consume This Natural Source of Protein.

To determine if eggs are safe for you, I recommend you test it yourself.

Carbohydrates: Grains, Beans and Legumes

Some health experts who advocate low-carb diets claim we should avoid carbs like beans, grains, and legumes.

Although some claim primitive man didn't eat carbs in the first place, recent evidence suggests that tubers, which are a type of carb, were consumed regularly in ancient times.

Many of today's carbs are made from highly-processed, denatured grains, such as white flours (e.g. breads, cakes and muffins), cookies, and other baked goods. High-temperature processing of grains (e.g. rice cakes, packaged cereals) is used to extrude these grains. These chemicals are dangerous for the body. You are left with an inedible starch, contaminated with chemicals from agribiz agriculture.

What about carbs other than whole grains? Although whole grains are full of nutrients, the problem with them today, even organic, is the high levels of phytic acid. These anti-nutrients, also known as phytotates, are hard to digest and can deplete your body's valuable minerals such as calcium, iron and magnesium. For more information, see Chapter 3.

It is important to get rid of the phytic acid from carbohydrates. This is very easy. For dinner that night, soak the rice overnight. Then rinse it, add some salt to taste, and then cook. Unsoaked grains will take half the time to cook. You may not feel the effects of poor preparation if carbs aren't a large part of your diet. It is best to soak any foods that contain phytic acid.

Low-carb or no-carb diets can be extreme. It is important to properly prepare carbohydrates and use whole grains, not devitalized processed ones. This simple step is crucial to reap the many benefits found in whole grains, beans, nuts and seeds.

Whole carbohydrate properly prepared can provide rich minerals, nutrients, and are delicious to eat. To make them more digestible and delicious, you can add organic butter or other good saturated fats.

Avoid extruded grains products made from whole grains such as rice cakes, flaked, and puffed cereals. They contain the highest levels of phytates, due to high-temperature processing.

Gluten in grains is a common allergy for many people. If you're one of these people, you can try soaking your flour or grain to see if it works better with phytate reduced breads. Gluten and phytates could be the culprit, or a combination of both.

To test whether you are able to tolerate gluten-reduced breads, you can do so personally. Making your own bread from fresh-ground flour and properly soaking it can help you digest previously intolerant grain products. Some of the older grains, such as kamut, are also available.

The Whole Grains Council website has some great information about whole grains.

> amaranth

> barley

> buckwheat

> corn, whole cornmeal and popcorn

> millet

> Oats, also known as oatmeal

> quinoa

> Rice, brown and colored rice

> rye

> sorghum (also known as milo)

> teff

> triticale

> wheat, including varieties like emmer, farro and einkorn as well as durum, kamut and forms such bulgur, cracked wheat, and wheat berries

> wild rice

NOTE: Before you start any recipe, make sure to follow the phytic Acid Reducing Soaking Procedures.

Ezekiel Cereals are a great breakfast cereal. They replace high-heat extruded puffs and flakes that increase the anti-nutrient phytotic acid. Ezekiel Cereals do not use high-heat extrusion. The company sprouts the grains in order to reduce phytates. They then slow cook them at a low heat to preserve nutrients. These grains are packed with a delicious crunch.

To further reduce the phytates in your beans and legumes, you can add a piece of kombu seaweed when cooking them. The kombu and the soaking both reduce flatulence (farting).

Soy

Soybeans contain high levels of phytates. To increase digestibility and nutrient absorption, they must be properly soaked and fermented. Soy is controversial. While some claim it has many health benefits, others warn about its potential dangers. I would only eat soy in its fermented form (like tempeh or traditional tamari) and avoid soy milk, tofu, and other products made with soy, especially commercial varieties that almost always contain GMOs.

These products can easily be tested in your home so that you are confident they are safe to eat.

The Cornucopia Institute -Organic Soy Scorecard lists the top soy producers. I will only eat products with ratings of 4 or 5 stars, and only products that have been fermented or soaked.

Learn more about the dangers of soy here: Are Soy Products Healthy?

<u>Soy Dangers Summarized</u>

Here's a breakdown of all the benefits of high-quality carbs (i.e. beans, legumes, and grains): The World's Best Foods.

Bread

A final note about phytates: If you love fresh bread, there is no better way than to grind the flour from whole grains. Traditions grind their grain fresh. This ensures that the flour is always fresh and doesn't lose vitamins or go rancid from being left out. Whole wheat flours should be refrigerated. Fresh grinding also has the added benefit of a great taste. So much better!

Here's how I use wheat. Here's my pancake and sourdough recipes:

My spring organic wheat berries are hand-ground into flour. This preserves the maximum nutritional value. I sometimes add 10-15% ryeberries and kamut to reduce the phytates in other grains. Kamut and Rye berries are rich in phytase, so they perform the phytate reduction trick when they're soaked.

Then I add water to the mixture and then mix in some whey. This is a tablespoon of yogurt or lemon juice. Let it sit on the counter for at least an hour. I drain the excess water, which contains phytates.

To make pancakes, I use 1/4 to 1/2 teaspoon baking soda or non-aluminum baking flour, and about a tablespoon of butter or olive oil. This stage will result in pancakes that are very thin. Use ghee or coconut oil to fry the pancakes in a cast iron skillet.

I usually make enough flour to have plenty of soaked flour. I save about half the flour for sourdough bread, and I use the rest to make pancakes. You can also use a starter sourdough to make the pancakes. Let it rest in a warm place for up to half a day until it develops a yeasty aroma. Next, drain any excess water.

I grind some more flour and then add it to the mixture with some sea salt. The dough is formed into a ball and kneaded for five minutes. Finally, place the dough in a bowl with damp cheesecloth. For a delicious breakfast or lunch, I cut some dough and make chapattis from it. The rest of dough is left to rise in the bowl for a few more hours. After that, I knead the dough for five minutes. Then, I place it in an oil bread pan to rise once more. After it has risen, I have sourdough bread that is ready to bake at 350° for 35-40 minutes or until it makes a hollow sound when it's tapped on top.

This bread is unique in taste and nutrition. When you are ready to eat it, add lots of butter! Toasting it gives it the best flavor. This method of preparing wheat may be acceptable for people with gluten sensitivities, as the gluten has already been pre-digested through the soaking and souring. To find out, test it.

Here's another easy recipe for whole grains such as wheat. Let them soak as previously described and then cook them whole just like rice. This article is from Scientific American:

> *Bread made with 80 percent whole-wheat kernels absorbs much*
> *slower than bread made from whole-wheat flour. The body*
> *must first break down the outer bran in order to digest the germ*
> *and inner endosperm. These metabolic brakes are often not*
> *provided by ground grains.*

Presoaking grains in water will lower their phytic acid levels and increase digestion. Saturated fats such as butter can also slow down digestion. Whole grains such as organic wheat are the best way to eat healthily.

Meat

Let's look closer at meat. Today's meat is so different from the natural meats of years past that it has become a dangerous food laden with omega-6 fats.

In order to increase the milk production and weight of livestock, it is possible to feed grains to them instead of grazing them. It created a highly lucrative industry.

Consumers have received meat and dairy products containing hormones, antibiotics, and an imbalanced ratio of omega-6 to Omega-3. These foods are a major contributor to the development of chronic diseases such as diabetes, heart disease, cancer, and other chronic conditions like allergies.

We eat poison! Our governments and industries have provided us with the lowest quality, cheapest food available without any concern for our health.

All that bad food is grade A (A should stand for "awful") It is a tragedy what has happened to our food supply. Hey, your nose never lies. You've probably driven past a factory cow farm or pig farm. It is horrible! You think food is healthy? Bring it on!

The key reason for the dramatic rise in Western prostate conditions including prostate cancer is likely to be hormonal imbalance. What causes this hormonal shift? It is considered a normal consequence of aging according to doctors. Alternative doctors often blame high fat, high milk and high-meat diets for the problem.

It is not all of the above. It is actually the altered nature of the meat, which is grain that has been fed antibiotics and growth hormones to alter once-healthy animal meat into toxic food.

Many people can feel upset by meat, particularly vegetarians and vegans. Because I was one for many decades, I understand!

You can test YES to high-quality, grass-fed organic meat by eating small slabs of meat and some fat. This will ensure that it is healthy for your health. These are some additional guidelines:

> Only eat grass-fed, free roaming, pastured meats. New Zealand lamb cannot be raised on pasture. It is widely available.

> You should avoid commercial toxic meat. It is dangerous due to the feeds used, and the toxins, estrogens and antibiotics that have accumulated in it.

Although organic grain-fed beef is better than conventional meat products, it still has an insufficient ratio of omega-6s and omega-3s. This is due to the fact that the cattle were fed grain, an unnatural food source even though organic!

The best meat comes from grass-fed cattle. Grass-fed cattle produce meat that has higher levels of beneficial omega-3 fatty acid and lower levels omega-6 fatty acid than those fed grain. Beef from grass-fed cattle is higher in betacarotene and other B vitamins, such as calcium, magnesium, vitamin E, potassium, and certain B vitamins. It also contains beneficial conjugated Linoleic Acid (CLA), which has anti-cancer properties.

> You are good for saturated fat! Consume meat with saturated fats, not lean meats. It's not high-quality protein, but it's protein with a lot of saturated fat. Weston A. has a lot of literature. Take a look at the literature from Weston A. Price Foundation to make your own decision.

Reduce the amount of meat you eat. For meat portion sizes, eat a portion that is smaller than your middle finger and fits in your palm. To determine if your palm-sized portion is appropriate, you can test it yourself.

> You can eat organ meats such as liver from time-to-time.

> Avoid high-temperature cooking. Ideal choices are stews, slow-roasted meats and lightly sauteed foods, as well as soups.

> Most prepared meats (i.e., sausages, etc.) Most prepared meats (e.g., sausages etc.) contain preservatives and toxins. These additives are the problem, and they are magnified by unhealthy meat.

Avoid barbecue meats. Charring causes carcinogens which are not good for the prostate!

You just have to have barbecued meat? Is the smell just too strong? Here's a compromise: Sometimes, you can lower the toxins. Don't be too generous! The compounds known as heterocyclic aminos (HCA) are a major cause of prostate cancer. They can be caused by grilling.

A new study has shown that meat marinated in herbs can dramatically reduce the amount of HCAs.

They marinated the steaks in three types of marinades for an hour and then grilled them at 400°F for five minutes each side. The marinade was not necessary for grilling steaks. Amazingly, steaks marinated with a "Caribbean mix" (thyme, red pepper, allspice and rosemary) showed an 88 percent decrease in HCAs. A herb marinade containing oregano and basil, onion, parsley and red pepper resulted in a 72 percent reduction. A third marinade containing paprika and red pepper, as well as garlic, onions, black pepper, and oregano, brought about a 57 per cent reduction.

Marinated Meats Less Toxic by J. Barron,
www.jonbarron.org/article/marinated-meats-less-toxic

Flare-ups due to burning fat are still a danger. Cook at the lowest temperature possible. Barbecue should be reserved for special occasions and not for regular use. You can also marinate your meat in vinegar or acidic lemon juice.

These articles provide a detailed review of primitive and traditional diets around the globe, as well as conclusions about saturated fats, meat and a balanced whole-foods diet:

Ancient Dietary Wisdom to Tomorrow's Children

<u>Characteristics of Traditional Diets</u>

What is wrong with "Politically Correct Nutrition"?

This book explains why grass fed meat is the best! The

Surprising Benefits from Grass Fed Meats, Eggs, and Dairy Products

This article will help you understand the differences between organic and grass-fed meat.

Dairy

Dairy is a controversial food, just like fats and meat. There are strong opinions, even among holistic health professionals. Dairy is an essential food according to conventional nutritionists. Others may blame dairy for your problems, and they might be right!

Today's dairy industry is facing the same fate as meat and fats. Modern agricultural practices and regulations have made once-healthy food a disease-generating toxin.

Modern dairy practices are the same as those that plague meat: unnatural feeds like grains, cramped quarters, modern feedlots, and pesticide-ridden food have all caused havoc on milk products, and the people who consume them. You have dairy products that are no longer suitable for human consumption if you add homogenization and pasteurization.

Yes, you can eat it. But over time, the critics of dairy products will be proven right. It's not that dairy products are bad food per se, as many pundits assert, but rather because of the way we treat these foods.

My view on dairy: Some people are able to digest milk easily due to their genetic heritage, while others (e.g. Asians) can have trouble with dairy, especially non-pasteurized varieties.

Start slow if you are new to dairy. You should first test and retest (see Chapter 10), the various dairy products that you select. Raw dairy products are much more tolerant and less reactive than those who have previously had issues with dairy. Some raw cheeses, butter, and ghees do not contain lactose. Pasteurization may cause sensitivities/allergies in some people.

Milk and Pasteurization

Ultrapasteurized milk is the majority of milk, even organic. Ultrapasteurization refers to heating milk to at least 280°F. This is well above the boiling point of 212°F. This is done to prolong the shelf life of milk and to kill germs that may have grown in unsanitary conditions such as cramped quarters.

It is not well-known what the ultra-pasteurization process does to the natural enzymes found in milk, and how it affects the human body. The Weston A. The Weston A:

> Ultrapasteurization and pasteurization are both rapid heat treatments that flatten molecules, making it impossible for enzymes to do their job. These proteins can get into the bloodstream, which is a common occurrence in people with 'leaky stomach'. This condition can be caused by consumption of processed milk products. The body then perceives them as foreign proteins and launches an immune response. This can lead to a chronically stressed immune system, and less energy for growth and repair.

> Ultra-Pasteurized milk by L. J. Forristal

www.westonaprice.org/modern-foods/ultra-pasteurized-milk

You can't forget about the harmful effects of milk packaging. You can also read on the same site about the dangers and risks associated with this harmful process as well as the hazards of plastic containers, which are very common in today's world.

> The processing of ultra-high-temperature processed milk can cause health problems and palatability issues. However, the packaging of the milk is equally important: both the aseptic containers and the plastic

containers. The milk can be contaminated by phthalates or other hormone disrupting chemicals (EDC).

Ultra-Pasteurized milk by L. J. Forristal

www.westonaprice.org/modern-foods/ultra-pasteurized-milk

Normal pasteurization heats milk to 250°F and applies pressure. It is perhaps a little better than ultra-pasteurized, but it is still not a healthy or whole food.

Andreas Moritz, Timeless Secrets of Health and Rejuvenation, also discusses the problems associated with milk pasteurization:

> *After milk has been pasteurized or ultra-heated, the natural enzyme population of the milk is destroyed. The enzymes are still needed to make the nutrients in the milk available to the cells. Six months after their birth, calves that were fed pasteurized cow's milk die. Imagine the chaos that must be happening in the tiny intestines of babies who are fed pasteurized milk or sterilized formula milk. These babies are more likely to have colic, be bloated, chubby, get sick frequently, cry often, and become restless.*

The healthiest milk is organic, raw milk from grass-fed cattle. This is the dairy of old. If milking and dairy facilities have been cleaned thoroughly, it is safe and extremely nutritious.

> *It has been shown that raw milk can prevent scurvy and other illnesses such as the flu, TB, or allergies. Raw milk, which is whole and pasteurized, contains essential fat-soluble vitamins A, D, and K2 as well as B12, C, calcium and iron. This can be easily utilized by the body. Most of these nutrients are lost when milk is pasteurized. Restricted protein, calcium, and D vitamins are lost and not absorbed well. In some cases, allergic reactions may develop as the body attacks what it*

Read more at these links: What is Real Milk?

Dairy Un-Forbidden - Discover the Virtues Of Raw Milk

Scientists Confirm Raw Milk Safe

Finally, I found raw milk that I was able to test. Both commercial milk and organic pasteurized milk (including yogurts from most brands) test NO. However, raw milk and raw milk yogurt at 180 degrees F have a YES result. My tongue doesn't have a white coating when I drink raw milk, which indicates poor digestion. My tongue develops a white coating from pasteurized milk by morning.

There were also delicious raw milk cheeses that I found at the health food shop. I also tested YES to raw milk cheese, while all other pasteurized cheeses (including organic) were NOs.

Moritz described how boiling milk can have a beneficial effect in Timeless Secrets of Health and Rejuvenation. It is important to distinguish between slow boiling at a lower temperature (180deg to212degF) and rapid heating under pressure to temperatures of 250deg to 220degF for pasteurization. These are completely different processes. Traditional cultures have been slow boiling at lower temperatures for many years.

The beneficial effect of boiling fresh, unpasteurized milk before drinking is apparent. Boiling milk protein breaks down into amino acids, making it easier to absorb and digest. This could be why East Indians boil their milk before using it. They are also aware that milk can have adverse effects if it is reduced in fat.

Moritz gives us a brief overview of digestibility and milk temperatures:

It is difficult to digest cold milk. The cold milk can cause nerve endings to become 'numb' or insensitive when it touches the warm stomach lining. Cells will also shrink or tighten as a result. This causes the production of gastric juices to stop digesting milk protein. Even worse, the cold milk can cause allergies by leaving some proteins unabsorbed. To be active on food enzymes, they need to be at a certain temperature. If the temperature is too low, the proteins won't be broken down properly. This can lead to intense irritation to the mucus membrane.

Although organic dairy products are superior to commercial dairy products, pasteurization can still cause problems.

Pasteurization destroys important enzymes such as lactase, which can cause many people to have difficulty digesting milk. Vitamins (like A, C, and B6 are reduced and fragile milk proteins transform from being health-promoting to unnatural amino acids configurations that can actually harm your health. Pasteurization can also promote pathogens, rather than protect you from them. . .

Pasteurization can cause allergic reactions and other problems in milk's physical structure.

Mainstream Nutrition by Dr.

Mercola,
articles.mercola.com/sites/articles/archive/2013/02/25/mainstreamnutrition-biggest-lies.aspx

Homogenized milk refers to a process that prevents fat from seperating from the milk. The milk is more difficult to digest when homogenization is performed under high pressure and with higher heat. Many people are allergic to this milk.

Raw milk and dairy are completely natural, healthy foods that can be used in place of all processed versions. You can try raw milk!

Click here to see where you can find raw milk and real cheese. You should also try raw goat milk or sheep milk as well as cheeses.

Raw milk can also be found in cow share programs, farmers and right here at the Raw Milk Institute.

Many of the arguments against raw milk are false, by the way. Pasteurization was created because New York's early 1900s growers used cramped quarters. The only way to fix the unsafe conditions was to promote pasteurization, rather than providing safe sanitary conditions for happy cows.

Harvard University has released a new study that shows pasteurized milk products from factory farms can cause hormone-dependent cancers. Concentrated animal feeding operations (CAFO), a method of raising cows on factory farms, produces milk with high levels of estrogen sulfate. This estrogen compound is linked to breast, testicular and prostate cancers.

Harvard Study: Pasteurized milk from industrial dairies linked to

Cancer by J. Benson,

Raw dairy, such as yogurt or milk, was mentioned earlier in the book. Raw foods do not include raw dairy.

Nuts and Seeds

These wonderful healthy foods are great, but there is a catch. Like grains and beans, nuts, seeds and legumes contain high amounts of the antinutrient phytic, along with enzyme inhibitors, which can cause mild to severe allergic reactions. This is in addition the mineral binding action that phytic acids has, thereby reducing the body's mineral content and the prostate. (See Chapter 3: Anti-Nutrients).

It was my unnoticed response to the disease that slowly worsened. I used to eat a lot of nuts and nut butters. My prostate condition progressed and I became more sensitive to nuts. I eventually got blocked from all the nuts and would not let out any pee. I was shut down by nuts such as cashews, nuts of Brazil, nuts of Brazil, nuts of Brazil, nuts from Brazil, nuts from Brazil, nuts from Brazil, nuts and nuts from walnuts. It's not fun.

Now I understand why. It was due to the enzyme inhibitors and the phytates. These natural ingredients protect the nut against predators as it grows and prevents premature sprouting. To be safe and easy to digest, nuts must be reduced in phytate. This can be done by soaking overnight in warm water and salt, then drying in your oven at 150°C. These make them taste even better and are crunchier. It is also possible to soak the seeds in water and then sprout them.

You can eat small amounts of nuts or seeds if you don't have any allergies and have no other conditions. If you eat nuts, seeds, nut milks such as almond milk or nut butters regularly, it is best to either make them yourself or find ones that have been prepared for you. These are becoming more common in health food shops.

Many nutrients found in nuts are good for the prostate. Almonds are the easiest to digest, especially if they are soaked overnight and then dried or roasted afterward. Brazil nuts and walnuts can both reduce prostate size and help with the growth of prostate cancer. For maximum bioavailability and phytate reduction, soak the nuts in water and then dry them.

> *The data suggests that walnuts can be used on a regular basis to delay, prevent, or delay certain types of cancer, such as breast and prostate. The health benefits of walnuts include a lower incidence of heart disease, cognitive decline and men's reproductive health. They also optimize blood lipids, weight management, and the optimization of many other forms of cancer. . . . Two ounces of water daily can prevent many chronic diseases.*

> *J. Phillip: A handful of walnuts every day can slow or prevent prostate cancer growth*

http://www.naturalnews.com/041343_walnuts_prostate_cancer_breast.ht

Walnuts can be soaked in warm saltwater for between 4-8 hours, and dried in a toaster oven at 130-150°F until they become crunchy.

To test nuts, personally test them. After drying and soaking, a NO response may become a YES. Even if the answer is YES, you should still include soaking to get the maximum benefit and minimize reaction. Non-organic nuts should be avoided. California almonds have been sprayed and walnuts are irradiated. If you have allergies to nuts, it is worth checking how many nuts you should eat each day. Avoid eating too many nuts, especially Brazil nuts.

Cracked nuts can easily go rancid so be careful. Nut butters can cause allergic reactions. Avoid mixed nuts and dried fruits that are packaged. Avoid canned, packed, and processed commercial nuts.

Pumpkin seeds contain high amounts of phytic acids and should be soaked. Pumpkin seeds and pumpkin seed butter are said to have a zinc content that can help the prostate. Regular consumption of pumpkin seeds is more harmful than helpful unless the phytic acid in them is reduced through soaking.

The phytic acid level in sesame seeds is very high, so it is the best food to remove the hull. They were all removed by traditional cultures. It is better to buy white, not unhulled brown--sesame seed.

I used to eat a lot of sesame seed, most with the hull. I used to eat sesame butter, gomasio (roasted sesame seed with salt), and ground seeds in smoothies. After eating sesame seeds one night, I experienced a reaction in my prostate. The seeds had blocked my pee tube. . . misery. I tested all my food the next morning and found the culprit: sesame seeds!

Tahini has no hulls and is therefore a great sesame seed product. However, sesame oil found in health food shops is made with sesame oils with the hulls still on (and many phytates). Avoid sesame butter.

Flax and chia seeds are two other great seeds. They are both superfoods. However, I have experienced reactions to them. It is important to eat healthy seeds and nuts in moderation. It is strongly recommended to soak the toxins in order to reduce them.

For more information on nuts and seeds high nutrient content, visit The World's Healthiest Foods.

Fruits and Vegetables

It is best to eat as many fruits and vegetables as possible, paying close attention to the seasons and where they were grown. These foods are more nutritious and more vital because they are picked at full ripeness.

It is important to test foods from the tropics in your own home (see Chapter 10), to determine if they are suitable for northern climates in the middle of winter. In our temperate climates, tropical fruits are not suitable for daily consumption, especially in winter.

You will experience fewer reactions if you are healthier. You'll be able to eat many different foods without any problems. Testing is necessary if you are in an extremely critical situation. Your body is rebuilding and can't deal with less than ideal inputs.

This is what I'm sure you didn't know about sweet potatoes, especially the red-fleshed ones:

> *They were ranked #1 in nutrition by the Center for Science in the Public Interest, as they provide a great source of complex carbohydrates, dietary fiber, natural sweeteners, protein, carotenoids and vitamin C.*

> *Nine Reasons to Eat More Sweet Potatoes by E. Walling,*
> *www.naturalnews.com/031543_sweet_potatoes_minerals.html*

Local produce should be organically grown and not sprayed. This article will provide you with a perspective on personal and environmental health. Local and organic food farming: Here's how to get the Gold Standard.

Learn to Read Labels on Produce

Produces will have a series number on them, like an orange. Usually, there are five numbers in a row (e.g. 94046). You can find out how the produce was grown by looking at the first number:

#9 = Organic (selenium- and nutrient-rich)

GMO foods (genetically modified enzymes and genes) are also available.

#8 = Containing pesticides or herbicides

#4 = Conventional produce (contains herbicides and pesticides).

You can eat a variety of fruits, vegetables and raw foods every day. The following factors will influence the amount of raw food you eat: where you live, how much sunlight you get, your current season, your current digestion strength (cooked is better for most foods if your digestion is compromised as most people do), the results of your personal tests (see Chapter 10).

Don't assume you can eat all fruits and vegetables because they are naturally delicious. Unknown reactions, or slow weakness from some vegetables and fruits can occur if you have a medical condition. It was so surprising to me that even my own beet and kale leaves can cause reactions!

To find local produce growers, use the Farmigo link. Mercola also offers information about local growers.

Nightshade Vegetables

Nightshade vegetables include tomatoes, bell peppers, eggplants, potatoes, and eggplants. Some of these vegetables can cause reactions in sensitive eaters. These include digestive problems, prostate reactions, arthritis, rheumatism and nervous system reactions.

These vegetables contain harmful glycoalkaloids. These toxins are high in the green parts of potatoes, and their eyes. Many people are unaware that they are allergic to tomatoes. These foods can contain solanine, which can cause severe reactions. Nightshades should be tested frequently and stopped if you have an allergic reaction, at the very least, for a short time.

To help them digest properly, it's best to eat potatoes with lots of butter.

Oxalate Vegetables

High amounts of oxalic acids are found in chives, parsley, Swiss chard and beet leaves. The oxalic acid forms urinary stones when it binds to minerals such as calcium and iron. This can easily cause irritation of the prostate. You should not eat oxalate vegetables unless you have tested positive.

Sweeteners

Because sugars are food for cancer cells, they can be linked to the growth of cancer cells. This includes prostate cancer. Sugars can cause problems with digestion and obesity, especially when they are combined with refined white carbohydrates.

The amount of sugar consumed has gone up dramatically. Our ancestors only ate one tablespoon of unprocessed sugar per day; we now consume more than a cup per day, mostly from highly refined sugars like white sugar and worse, high fructose corn syrup. Imagine the people at the top of the food chain eating more than the average.

Most prepared foods contain sugar. High fructose corn syrup is a highly refined sweetener that can be even more dangerous than sugar cane. For more information, see this article: The murky world of high-fructose corn syrup.

High fructose corn syrup and fructose corn sugar (HFCS) are dangerous sweeteners that can cause metabolic syndrome, diabetes and cardiovascular disease. They can be found in processed foods as well as fast food. For more information, see this article: Diabetes Obesity Metabolism Journal Article.

You can also see Dr. Robert Lustig's YouTube video Sugar: The Bitter truth, which explains the harm caused by fructose. Fructose, one of the main causes of obesity, is also a factor.

High fructose corn syrup, which is found in many fast food and supermarket foods, poses another danger. GMO corn is used to grow most of the syrup. A recent large-scale study in France found that genetically engineered foods caused severe cancerous lesion in rats (see Chapter 3 section on toxins).

Fruit juices are better than regular sugar, so avoid them. Orange juice contains almost the same amount of sugar as Coke. You can dilute fruit juices with water 4 to 1. That's 4 units water to 1 juice. You can also eat whole fruits, as the fiber helps to reduce fructose.

Some pundits claim that Agave nectar, or syrup, is a healthier sugar than sugar. It is actually a super-condensed fructose syrup that lacks virtually any nutrient value. You can read more about Agave here: Marketing triumphs over truth.

Stevia is a safer alternative. Many of the reduced versions are potentially dangerous. Learn more. You can only test it yourself to find out. Every time I get a No.

Artificial sweeteners don't make it any better and can even be worse. They are low in calories, so people use them. They can actually increase sugar cravings. The chemicals can also cause weight gain because they are not good for your body. You're just trading one bad habit for another. Learn all about artificial sweeteners and their dangers here: Sugar-Free Blues.

Healthy Sugar Alternatives

> Maple syrup is real maple syrup, not imitation. The darker the maple syrup, the greater its nutrients. Grade B, C or #2 (different grading system). Maple syrup is rich in potassium, calcium, and nutritionally important amounts of zinc as well as manganese and manganese. Zinc is an important prostate mineral. Pure maple syrup, which is rich and dark organically produced, can be used in moderation. If you don't find it in your local grocery store, you can buy organic maple syrup here.

Raw honey, unfiltered, the best. Darker honey, just like maple syrup, has more trace elements. Cooking honey can destroy its healthy enzymes. Use only non-cooking recipes.

> Molasses

> Sucanat and Rapadura: Dehydrated sugarcane juice

> Date sugar

> Organic Coconut Sugar

Many people are addicted sugar and unknowingly to the addictive additives found in processed foods. Your cravings will begin to diminish if you eat high-quality saturated fats like the ones I mentioned earlier. Replace toxic sugars with healthier alternatives. Reduce the amount you consume. Moderation is key when it comes to sweeteners and desserts. A maximum of one to two tablespoons per day is sufficient.

Water

Water is the most important food after air. It heals and harms. Start paying more attention to how the water you consume and drink in beverages and your cooking!

Most tap water in cities contains chlorine, fluoride, and residues from all kinds of toxic chemicals. Tap water is often not suitable for human consumption. Bottled water is not as good.

Most bottled water is the same as basic tap water. However, it does cost 50 to 100 times more per gallon that basic tap water. Worse, plastic water bottles can leach xenoestrogenic chemicals. These chemicals can disrupt the hormonal balance of the body. BPA (bisphenol A) is one example. It is linked to neurodevelopmental issues in children. BPA can cause premature puberty in boys and lead to breast growth in girls. BPA has been linked to prostate, breast, uterine and ovarian cancers.

Bottled Water is Hazardous to You and Our World by Dr. D. Jockers, www.naturalnews.com/032744_bottled_water_environment.html Look at this chart about bottled water vs. tap water.

A water purifier is the best solution. There are many choices. Brita countertop units will remove chlorine, but not other contaminants. Aquasana filters are highly rated and inexpensive. They can be used at the sink as well as for the entire house.

A water distiller is my preference. Some health experts claim that distilled water can cause mineral loss. Water has very little minerals. You can get them from your food. To add minerals back to the water and revitalize it, I add quarter teaspoon of sea salt per gallon to my distilled water.

I prefer distillers with a stainless steel chamber, a glass collection container, and not one made of plastic. Waterwise's smallest unit is the Waterwise 4000. This distiller is made in America and can distill a gallon of water in approximately 3-4 hours. They are also available on Amazon.com, though beware of plastic models. Water distillers at Amazon.com.

Berkey Water Filters is another high-rated water filter that comes in many sizes, both for your home and travel.

Vitamin C is a cheap way to eliminate chlorine from your bath water. This is especially useful if your intention is to relax in the tub without the irritation caused by chlorine.

When we shower and bathe, our bodies absorb chlorine and other heavy metals. Your toxic load will increase over time. There are simple, inexpensive devices you can use to filter your water. These items are available at Amazon:

Bath Dechlorinators

Whole-House Chlorine Water Filters

Waterwise has a showerhead that is simple, affordable and very effective. They say this:

Showerwise helps to reduce inhalation of vapors as well as the absorption of chemicals. It effectively removes chlorine and other contaminants. . . Also, it controls many types of bacteria such as algae, fungi, and mold.

Waterwise Deluxe Showerwise Filtration System

It is important to test your water to make sure it is safest for you. You can ask your friend or relative for help in determining the best filter system. To find the best bottled water, I test it in supermarkets. Each time I do this, the distilled winner is mine.

How much water should you drink?

According to most health experts, we should consume at least 8 cups (8 oz.) of water per day. per cup). According to them, most people are chronically dehydrated and require more water to maintain their internal organs. They say that 70% of our bodies is water so it is vital to drink enough.

Although it is true that we may be dehydrated, this could also be due to our poor diet, which is laden with too much salt and toxins. This is where you need to start making changes.

It is recommended to flush out the toxins with water. However, this may only add to the problem:

Drinking a lot of water during the day can cause stomach acid to become diluted. This can lead to acid reflux, as well as all the other problems discussed. It is possible to have digestive problems due to excessive water intake.

Over-consuming water can cause constipation, paradoxically. If you consume too much water in addition to high-fiber foods, fibrous foods can swell and ferment in your intestinal tract. This can lead to gas, bloating, and other unpleasant digestive symptoms. The increased mass could be too large for the body to handle.

People who drink large amounts of water will not only lower their stomach acid, but also have a reduced ability to digest and absorb nutrients. This can lead to malnutrition over time.

Acid Reflux: A Red Flag by K. Pirtle,
www.westonaprice.org/digestivedisorders/acid-reflux-a-red-flag

Roger Mason echoes this view. Although I disagree with some parts of Mason's book, it makes sense to me:

Many people are surprised to hear that you should only drink when you feel thirsty. Only drink when you feel the need. False thirst for water is not the same as false hunger for food. Many nutritionists recommend drinking quarts of water every day, regardless of whether you feel thirsty. These people claim that we are 'dehydrated'. This is a false statement. This drink-asmuch-as-you-can theory is very harmful--'drink eight glasses a day'.

Proponents believe that your kidneys can be flushed out like sewer pipes. The opposite is true. Your kidneys work less efficiently if you consume more. Your kidneys work differently from the plumbing system of your home. Your kidneys filter, absorb and diffuse water. They should not be overloaded. Too much liquid can overload your kidneys, making it impossible for them to perform the tasks they were designed to do. Too much water can cause cells to close and water that isn't filtered will be diverted to the large intestinale. The water is then sent to the bladder, where it will be eliminated without any treatment. Your body retains the toxins.

DO NOT DRINK IF YOU ARE NOT DESIRED. To show that there are many toxins in your urine, your urine shouldn't be cloudy. It should be clear and yellowish. It's very difficult to drink if you aren't thirsty. This is against our instincts. We shouldn't drink if we don't have to.

R. Mason: Zen Macrobiotics for Americans

Many water experts fail to account for factors such as climate, age and body size. Everyone seems to follow everyone else's advice, so we believe we should drink 8 glasses a day! You'd be surprised at how many people keep water bottles around, drinking blindly according to these guidelines.

A new study by CBC TV has disproved the ridiculous excess water drinking myth.

Some experts say you shouldn't drink water during meals. Drinking small amounts of water when you're thirsty can help digestion. Drinking water 15-20 minutes before or after meals is a good idea to avoid diluting the digestive juices. Avoid cold water. This is bad for the kidneys. What affects your prostate will also be harmful. The East doesn't drink cold water, but they do drink warm water.

Don't drink if you aren't thirsty. Dehydration can cause more harm than overhydration. It is important to have the right amount of fluids and water.

Water intoxication, also known as hyponatremia, refers to excessive water intake or bodily fluids. Extreme dilution can cause a variety of problems. Take a look at Wikipedia.

Observable symptoms of water intoxication: headache, personality changes, changes in behavior, confusion, irritability, and drowsiness. These are sometimes followed by difficulty breathing during exertion, muscle weakness, twitching, or cramping, nausea, vomiting, thirst, and a dulled ability to perceive and interpret sensory information. As the condition persists papillary and vital signs may result including bradycardia (fatigue, weakness, dizziness, light-headedness, fainting, chest discomfort, palpitations, or shortness of breath) and widened pulse pressure.

It goes on to describe even worse conditions that can happen from too much diluted fluids in the body.

So, dear reader, there goes the myth of drinking water all day long as being healthy!

How can you tell how many fluids are in your body (and this includes not just water but all your drinks, teas, coffees and liquid foods)?

Look at the color of your urine.

Too dark and you are dehydrated; too light (no color) = too hydrated. Balanced = a clear, yellow color.

Caffeinated Drinks

You will find lots of information both for and against caffeinated drinks, especially around coffee. Some researchers say caffeine is very healthy and others say just the opposite. A simple solution is to personally test the caffeinated drinks that you regularly consume. You will know right away. If you get a YES, then do not assume it means that you can drink as much as you want. Test again to find your optimum number of cups (see *Personal Testing* in Chapter 10). It's best to drink organic versions of coffee because of the toxins present in regular coffee. The same goes for caffeinated teas and chocolate (dark is best).

Many people recommend green tea for its health benefits. Green tea contains caffeine. Test that to see if it is okay for you and see if decaf green varieties are better. I still get a NO for green tea despite its supposed benefits.

Herbal Teas

You will find that many herbal teas can be troublesome for your prostate if you have a condition, so be careful and test often. Recently the teabags themselves have been found in many cases to contain toxins. So best to use loose teas and not those in bags.

Beer Wine and Liquor

Fermented beers can be a wonderful beverage, especially from small homemade batches or microbreweries. If you test YES, ensure that you drink the beer in moderation because hops contain estrogens, which is not a desirable input for your prostate except occasionally.

Try organic wines, as grapes are one of the most-sprayed foods. Personally test to see if you can drink wine, whether red or white, and how much.

Test any liquor you want. I find that there are some fine liquors I can drink a bit of on occasion without a reaction, but most times I get a NO response.

Lacto-Fermented Foods

Probiotics are live microorganisms in our foods and are proven to be beneficial to the digestive system. Probiotics improve the absorption of nutrients and promote a healthy immune system. This is a very important food group that helps digestion immensely.

It is the good bacteria and enzymes found in raw unpasteurized lactofermented foods like traditional yogurt, sauerkraut and pickles (without vinegars) that are not only tasty but also help prevent gas and irritable digestion, as well as many other benefits.

Today, many health gurus highly recommend adding all kinds of digestive enzymes in the form of supplements to your diet. There is also a trend to add enzymes like acidophilus in processed yogurts and other foods.

A far superior way to get probiotics is from traditional lacto-fermented foods. These foods have been used around the world in all cultures to preserve foods and to aid digestion. They do work wonders—I can vouch for that. The enzymes help digestion in the upper stomach where there are no digestive fluids and further aid digestion by providing lactic acid.

Lacto-fermented foods, such as natural yogurt, contain plentiful amounts of natural probiotics, which normalize the acidity of the stomach and do much more:

> *Like the fermentation of dairy products, preservation of vegetables and fruits by the process of lacto-fermentation has numerous advantages beyond those of simple preservation. The proliferation of lactobacilli in fermented vegetables enhances their digestibility and increases vitamin levels . . .*
>
> *These beneficial organisms produce numerous helpful enzymes as well as antibiotic and anticarcinogenic substances. Their main by-product, lactic acid, not only keeps vegetables and fruits in a state of perfect preservation but also promotes the growth of healthy flora throughout the intestine.*
>
> *Nourishing Traditions: The Cookbook that Challenges Politically Correct Nutrition and the Diet Dictocrats* by S. Fallon and M. Enig

Here is another wonderful book filled with simple recipes to brew all kinds of delicious fermented treats:

Wild Fermentation: The Flavor, Nutrition, and Craft of Live-Culture Foods

These lacto-fermented foods are great sources of probiotics and are ideal for daily eating at each meal—natural, unpasteurized versions without vinegars are the most potent:

> Yogurt

> Tamari

> Miso

> Tempeh

> Sauerkraut

> Buttermilk

> Kefir

> Cottage cheese

> Sourdough breads

> Pickles of all kinds

Use these natural forms of probiotics regularly and see the difference they make to your overall digestion. Always test first to ensure your compatibility, and start with very small amounts. Learn more about personal testing in Chapter 10.

> *Lacto-fermented beverages are ubiquitous in traditional cultures- from kefir beer in Africa to kvass and kombucha in Slavic regions. Lactofermented foods are artisanal products—instead of mass produced items preserved with vinegar and sugar—which taste delicious and confer many health benefits. They add valuable enzymes to the diet, and enhance digestibility and assimilation of everything we eat.*
>
> *Nasty, Brutish and Short?* by S. F. Morell,
> www.westonaprice.org/traditional-diets/nasty-brutish-short

Read more about the benefits of probiotics here:

California Dairy Research Foundation: US Probiotiocs

National Center for Complementary and Alternative Medicine: Oral Probiotics

You can get some wonderful cultured veggies here.

Probiotic supplements are highly promoted, but the above foods are the best way to go. If you can't eat them because of travel or other reasons, then in the short term, taking probiotic supplements may be useful.

If you are coming off a bad diet, then both lacto-fermented foods and probiotics would be beneficial. Always personally test these lacto-fermented foods to know if they are right for you and what quantities you should have daily. Sometimes therapeutic doses of probiotics can help a leaky gut. Increase your intake for a short while by increasing your dose by a factor of 2–5 times per day.

Always test to ensure you are not overdoing it. Keep in mind that your body's needs do change! I had too much lacto-fermented sauerkraut it seems, because after a few months of eating sauerkraut at every meal I started to react. I tested, got a NO response, and realized again that even the best of the best can turn into its opposite with excess use. Seems like I am a slow learner! Thank goodness for being able to personally test foods!

Salt

Commercial salt—sodium chloride—may have the same chemical structure as sea salt, but there is a world of difference. The trace elements in sea salt, not found in commercial salt, are invaluable in providing needed minerals in our diets. For example, sea salt is high in zinc, the crucial prostate mineral. It is an easy switch to make from commercial salts. It will also save you from taking an inferior mineral supplement and from being harmed by commercial salt.

Just as with wine, there are many differences amongst the sea salts you can find today: from the thick slightly grayish Celtic Sea salts to the reddish/pinkish Himalayan and Utah salts from buried seas millions of years ago and to the pure, sun-dried Antarctic sea salts on the beaches of South West Africa to the wonderful Hawaiian ones and many, many more!

The pinkish color that some sea salts have comes from the trace minerals in the sea salt. These are ideal salts for your diet. You will find the taste far superior to bland commercial bleached and refined salt or—worse yet—the low-sodium salt substitutes that industry claims are better for you.

Some commercial salt has iodine added back in, but sea salt already contains that and many more nutrient minerals—60 to 80 other needed nutrients, in fact.

Part of the process for refined salt, or commercial table salt, involves the use of aluminum, ferro cyanide and bleach. These are all toxic materials that your body takes in with refined, commercial salt. And because of that process, almost all the vital minerals that real, unrefined sea salt can offer are removed! One or two servings of refined salt won't send you to the grave. But continued almost daily use will avail you to the perils of aluminum toxicity. Ferro cyanide is listed by the EPA as a toxic material for human consumption. You are probably aware of the hazards to human health of chlorine, which is used to bleach the salt.

Why Himalayan Pink Crystal Salt is so Much Better for Your Health than Processed Table Salt by M. Adams,
www.naturalnews.com/028724_Himalayan_salt_sea.html

Read this article to learn about the different perils of refined salt: <u>Confront Salt Confusion</u>.

Discover the world of sea salt. Try different varieties of sea salts to discover your favorite and to vary the micro mineral content. It is easy to find in any health store. You can also find sea salt here at Amazon: <u>Sea Salt</u>.

Myth of Low Salt Diet

It has been drummed into our heads that a low salt diet is best for our health and our hearts. Here are 3 good articles to destroy that myth. Just make sure you eat high quality sea salt.

<u>The Salt of the Earth</u>

<u>Salt and Our Health</u>

<u>Scant Evidence</u>

Our earlier discussion on water and excess bodily fluids was not complete. The role of salt in helping to balance the body is equally important.
Use quality sea salt for real health benefits.

Herbs and Spices

These items add great variety and flavor to our foods. The problem is that many can be irritants, especially if they are used frequently or if they have become stale. The only way to know is to personally test them from time to time. Another danger is that people often keep them around too long; they lose their freshness and can go off, which causes even further reactions. A year is about the maximum time to keep herbs and spices unless refrigerated.

Also, some spices come irradiated, which creates a new danger to your health.

I have had severe reactions to many herbs and spices thinking they are used in such small amounts that it wouldn't matter. Then I wisened up (I am slow sometimes!) and started testing them. Eat safe. Check 'em out!

Ginger is a remarkable spice for killing prostate cancer cells and preventing it as well. For more information read *Benefits of Whole Ginger Extract in Prostate Cancer*. Use fresh ginger for best results.

Air

I call air a food because 10 to 20 times per minute we are consuming air. If the air is polluted you are at a health disadvantage. Make sure your home and car are protected if you live in air-polluted cities. Air purifiers with a negative ion generator can make a big difference. Read more at this site filled with expertise: Office and Home Air Purifiers.

How and When to Eat

Food is crucial for nourishing us. We need to learn to take more time than we are used to when it comes to preparing and eating whole foods. Food is your daily medicine and eating in a non-rushed manner is a good habit to develop.

Chewing more thoroughly than we are used to helps make the food much more digestible, so that we benefit from the high quality food choices we are now investing in.

In the Ayurvedic tradition, there are times that are thought best to eat that correspond with natural body biorhythms that enhance digestion. Those times are 8 am for breakfast, 12 noon for lunch and 6 pm for supper. Eating around these times (plus or minus an hour) is ideal. Avoid eating after 8 pm, as our digestive juices decline rapidly in the evening.

Get With It!

Adjust to the fact that quality food will cost more than cheapo foods that harm you. What price is your health? Are new technological and electronic devices more desirable than great health? Find ways to make your health the top of your priority list because without good health, your quality of life will be impacted greatly.

You can still save by buying in bulk, joining food coops and buying clubs, buying direct from the grower, attending local farmers markets and starting to grow your own food, even on a balcony. Take a look at <u>Journey to Forever's</u> website that has lots of resources for container gardening.

And now you can get all kinds of healthy foods delivered to your door inexpensively anywhere in the U.S. Check out:

<u>The Green Polka Dot Box</u>

It is a membership site that grows by referral. The benefits are truly amazing. They include:

> wholesale or deep discount pricing,

> free FedEx delivery,

> huge selection and major brands of organic foods,

> refrigerated, frozen and fresh organic veggies, >

personal care, household items and supplements, and

> natural pet and garden supplies.

Conclusion

> Eat widely across all food groups.

> Eat lacto-fermented foods to help you digest more.

> Eat slowly and chew well.

> If you want to drink while eating, sip rather than drink large quantities to aid your digestion.

> Limit desserts to one meal a day at most to lessen your addictions to sweets.

> Enjoy the rich tastes of natural wholesome foods!

Now that you know what the REAL foods are, read on to learn what the SUPER foods are.

Chapter 8: Superfoods

Superfoods are a group of foods that contain extra high amounts of beneficial nutrients. The list is subjective, as there is no official definition of what is and is not a superfood. Keep in mind, what may be a superfood for one could be harmful to another. The only way to know is to personally test each food you eat. That said, check some of these out: ghee, avocados and avocado oil, coconut oil, sauerkraut, miso, lemons and green superfoods.

Ghee

Ghee, also known as clarified butter, ideally made from the butter that comes from grass-fed cows, is a wonderful superfood. Ghee has a sweet buttery taste that adds both richness and flavor to your food. Ghee is basically butter with the milk protein and lactose taken out, leaving pure butter fat. Ghee has a higher burning point than butter, meaning you can cook it at much higher temperatures than butter without it burning. It's a great cooking oil.

Try some from <u>Pure Indian Foods</u>. They have several flavors, but I suggest you start with the plain version first.

Avocados and Avocado Oil

Avocados are a superfood delight and so delicious. They are filled with good fats that provide excellent anti-inflammatory benefits. Avocados contain:

> Phytosterols, including beta-sitosterol (found in Saw Palmetto)

> Carotenoid antioxidants

> Vitamins C and E

> Manganese

> Selenium

> Zinc

> Omega-3 fatty acids

Read more about avocados at <u>this website</u>.

Avocado oil has a very high burning point, so it is great for cooking and is delicious on salads. Get extra virgin, cold-pressed, organic varieties. It will cost more but <u>Avocado oil</u> is a superb, versatile, very healthy oil for more moderate use.

Want a potato chip made with healthy oils? Try these super yummy chips made with organic avocado oil: <u>Avocado Chilean Lime Chips by Good Health</u>.

As with all foods, remember not to overdo this oil. Since avocados are a tropical fruit, they are best eaten in moderation especially in winter if you test yes (see Chapter 10).

Coconut oil

This amazing oil, which is a saturated fat, is best in its extra virgin state. This means that like extra virgin olive oil, it has received the least amount of heat processing in order to preserve its optimum nutrient values. Coconut oil is perfect to cook with and to use in salads. It is also wonderful on your skin and hair. Read more here:

<u>Latest Studies on Coconut Oil</u>

<u>Latest Headlines on Coconut Health</u>

<u>The Many Benefits of Coconut Oil and Coconut Butter</u>

> *Coconut oil also helps to balance hormones, stabilize blood sugar levels and boost the cellular healing process. It is also known to stimulate the thyroid and reduce stress on the liver and pancreas. This increases metabolism which helps us burn fat far more effectively while stimulating clean sources of energy that make us feel terrific.*

> *Make Sure You Consume Enough of this Super Food* by Dr. D. Jockers, <u>www.naturalnews.com/030990_super_food_coconut_oil.html</u>

Coconut oil also provides effective and natural sun protection without having to use toxic chemicals in conventional sun block. Coconut oil guards against free radicals, providing added protection against skin cancer. Mix coconut oil with African Shea butter and aloe vera for a simple and harmless sun protection formula. This combination is also wonderful as a moisturizer for your skin and hair.

Coconut water kefir is a fermented beverage especially beneficial for gut problems such as candida overgrowth. This drink is hard to find but easy to make. Go here for tips: <u>Kefir Coconut Juice Recipe</u>. Coconut water is also an excellent drink to use during fasting because of its high nutritional content.

One caveat: coconut is tropical and some sensitive people may not tolerate much coconut oil or other coconut products. I am one of those. As always, test to know.

Miso

A traditional oriental food, miso is a lacto-fermented food packed with great taste and benefits. Traditionally, miso is aged 6 months to 2 years. If you go to Japanese restaurants, then you must be familiar with miso soup.

Unfortunately modern Japanese miso is now adulterated from its past traditional greatness, often highly processed and containing MSG. It is best to buy organic versions free from GMO soybeans and MSG.

> *Many studies have shown the health benefits of miso on humans and animals. Benefits include reduced risks of breast, lung, **prostate,** and colon cancer, and protection from radiation.*

> *Miso has a very alkalizing effect on the body and strengthens the immune system to combat infection. Its high antioxidant activity gives it anti-aging properties.*

> *Miso Soup: A Delicious Bowl Full of Health and Anti-Aging Benefits* by B. Minton, www.naturalnews.com/025519_health_anti-aging_soy.html

Miso often is made with rice or barley added to the soybeans during the fermentation process. I find the rice version (genmai miso) mild and delicious. You can find some here: Organic Miso.

Here is a very quick and simple way to use miso. Boil water, pour into a cup, add a teaspoon or more of miso and stir to dissolve. That's it—now you have a refreshing and uplifting drink with amazing health benefits.

Sauerkraut

This time-honored food, already talked about earlier, made from raw ingredients and sea salt is so beneficial for digestion. It can be an acquired taste for some people, so start slow with a small amount and use a young version rather than a longer-aged one.

Avoid pasteurized sauerkraut, as the pasteurization process destroys the beneficial nutrients in this superfood. Daily use will do wonders to your gut, so it is worth acquiring the taste. Start making your own since it is quick and easy to do. Here are some recipes for making your own sauerkraut and many more as this is THE cookbook to own: _Nourishing Traditions_.

Start with only a small teaspoon of sauerkraut and increase the amount slowly to limit reactions in sensitive people.

Lemons (and Limes)

Lemons contain vitamin C and bioflavonoids, plant derivatives with antioxidant and anti-inflammatory—as well as anti-cancer—properties. Lemons are a superb food for the prostate.

High in potassium, lemons affect the body's biochemistry and pH levels in a positive and powerful way. Astringent in nature, lemons have an overall alkalizing effect on the body, even though they are acidic before entering the body.

I like to use a little lemon juice in place of vinegar in salad dressings. You can add it to steamed veggies, soups, sauces, dips and even desserts. I add a bit when making applesauce.

Some mornings I start the day with some lemon squeezed into a cup of very hot water and mixed with a teaspoon of honey. Use unpasteurized honey. According to Ayurvedic practices, this drink is good for the liver and aids digestion and the immune system. I also switch honey for maple syrup for variety. Read more about lemons here: Lemons/Limes. Again test constantly. After all they are tropical foods. I only tolerate them for short time periods and then I react.

Green Superfoods

Greens or green superfoods are highly promoted as powders, juices and supplements. These include wheatgrass, chlorella, blue-green algae, barley greens, parsley powders, spirulina and more. Packed with natural nutrients, vitamins and minerals, green superfoods come highly recommended by many practitioners. I won't get into all the claims here because, in the final analysis, you will be the judge by personally testing to see if green superfoods are right for you.

Remember—it is what you can digest that counts not what the profile is of the food. Greens are raw foods and can be difficult to process.

Be careful with these greens, they can cause reactions in you and your prostate. If greens test positive for you, they can be beneficial in helping you rebuild after years of poor diet habits because of their high nutrient content. You can read more here:

The Natural News Store: search for "Green Superfoods"

Green Superfoods at Amazon

Pure Synergy® Superfood is a top-of-the-line green product I used to take. There is quite the story of where and how it is made.

It may be best to take a single green product rather than a mixture of many. You could test positive for an individual product, but a combination product could have something in it that disagrees with your system. So go to a health food store and start with single items to test. Then continue to test over time to ensure you do not end up with a negative reaction.

The simplest green product of all is liquid chlorophyll: World Organic Chlorophyll Liquid. It is the only green one that I have been able to tolerate well, perhaps because of its simplicity and compatibility with human blood.

Greens may be useful as part of a cleansing diet for the short term and not every day use. Over the long term, I would bet that most people will eventually test NO to them. So be careful.

The best green superfood of all may in fact be raw milk! That way you let the cow do the hard work of digesting the greens, something they are optimally designed to do. It is now my preferred way to have my greens because I test NO for almost all of them and always YES for raw milk and yogurt.

Other Superfoods

Many people have their own lists of foods that contain high concentrations of valuable nutrients. Superfoods are a far superior way to get a vitamin or mineral that you think you may be missing rather than taking a supplement. I will list some here:

> <u>Cod Liver Oil</u> is such an important food source. It is a potent food with vitamin D and omega-3s in an easy to absorb form that makes it so potent.

> <u>Manuka Honey</u>—there has been lots of research on honey products. This is medicinal honey.

> <u>Swedish Bitters</u> to balance all the tastes.

> <u>Evening Primrose Oil</u>, <u>Black Currant Oil</u> and <u>Borage Oil</u> are special, potent oils for very occasional use. Gamma Linoleic Acid (GLA), found in these oils, is an immune stimulator and anti-inflammatory

> <u>Kelp</u> has a high mineral content, especially iodine, which many people are deficient in. You can find powdered kelp with sea salt as a condiment that is quite tasty.

> <u>Wheat Germ Oil</u> is an excellent source of natural vitamin E that can be added to smoothies.

> Sprouts can be a powerhouse of concentrated nutrition. Soaking and then sprouting releases nutrients and decreases anti-nutrients like phytic acid in grains, nuts, beans and seeds. Sprouts are a great way of having fresh greens in the winter, bioavailable vitamins, minerals, amino acids, proteins, beneficial enzymes and phytochemicals. The only caveat is that you personally test them to ensure their compatibility as with any superfoods you eat. Sprouting is easy to do right in your kitchen. Get seeds at your local health food store or at Amazon: <u>Sprouting Seeds</u>.

Mushrooms

Certain mushrooms have powerful healing and prevention properties and, hence, can be deemed to be superfoods. These include shiitake, enokidake, maitake and oyster mushrooms. Ideally, get them fresh from large natural foods stores or Asian markets.

Mushrooms contain a host of antioxidants like selenium and immunity boosters like beta-glucans, which protect the body against invading organisms. Mushrooms contain cancer-fighting substances that protect against breast and prostate cancers. Mushrooms are best eaten cooked.

Allium Vegetables

These include garlic and onions. High consumption of these vegetables protects against stomach and prostate cancers.

Super Seeds

Seeds have healthy omega-3 fats and have minerals and vitamins our bodies need. Personally test these seed types before eating them, and then find the correct quantity. Often the best way to eat seeds is by grinding them first. I grind mine in a coffee grinder.

Chia Seeds

Organic chia seeds contain 15 times more magnesium than broccoli, 6 times more calcium than whole milk, 3 times more antioxidants than fresh blueberries, more fiber than flaxseed, plus more protein than soy and are extremely high in omega-3 fatty acids. It's fat though is not easy to convert into the usable forms of omega-3, EPA and DHA.

As with other seeds and nuts, to reduce phytates you may need to sprout and then dry the seeds before consuming them. You can find some organic varieties made from sprouted seeds. I still test negative for chia, perhaps because I used too much before I knew about personally testing foods and phytates. If you get a YES response when you test, remember to go slow to start and retest often.

Flaxseeds

Touted today by many as a superfood, flaxseeds can be highly beneficial, as can its oil because of its beneficial high omega 3s. The seeds like Chia, however, contain high levels of phytates and the oil also does not convert easily into the usable forms of omega-3, EPA and DHA. Best to make flax fresh grounded in your coffee grinder. If you use flax oil, it must be refrigerated to keep its potency. Add a teaspoon occasionally to your salads.

Pumpkin Seeds

Pumpkin seeds have been used in many cultures to treat BPH and prostatitis. They may also help with prostate cancer. Pumpkin seeds are rich in zinc, a mineral for prostate health.

Pumpkin seeds and their oil may be useful, but pumpkin seeds do contain phytates, so it is best to buy them whole and soak the seeds to reduce the phytic acid before eating them.

Pumpkin seeds are also available as a nut butter; I used to eat it often before I knew about the phytate anti-nutrient and had to stop when I had prostate reactions. I still test negative to pumpkin seeds, including its oil. So you know what to do now! Test for yourself to see if these seeds are good for you! (See *Personal Testing* in Chapter 10).

Antioxidants

This is a controversial subject with many health advocates proclaiming the benefits of taking antioxidants daily as a supplement. Although, some recent research suggests that over-indulging in antioxidants can have a harmful effect, this study refutes that claim: Study Citing Antioxidant Vitamin Risks Based On Flawed Methodology, Experts Argue.

The National Institutes of Health stated, "Antioxidants are substances that may prevent potentially disease-producing cell damage that can result from natural bodily processes and from exposure to certain chemicals." Antioxidants and Health: An Introduction

Here is a summary of the supposed benefits of antioxidants:

Studies over the last 20 years have shown that free radical fighters found in a certain group of nutrients, namely antioxidants, can protect against a great many free radical initiated diseases. Antioxidants extinguish free radicals!

Free Radicals cause oxidation in the blood. Once oxidation occurs, disease can result. Antioxidants keep free radicals from causing oxidation in the blood, thus neutralizing disease. Also, stress, chemical pollution, environmental pollution, and the normal aging process increase the demands put upon the immune system.

Studies indicate antioxidants do more than protect against free radicals; they also stimulate the immune system's response to help fight existing diseases.

Antioxidant Benefits and Antioxidant Formulas by Health and Nutrition, www.antioxidants.net/antioxidant-benefits

This next article lays out the specific ones that the author believes are the best (Acai, resveratrol, quercetin, pine tree bark, curcumin, lutein, zeaxanthin, lycopene, selenium, catalase, R-lipoic and humic/fulvic acid): The Vital Role of Antioxidants in Achieving Optimum Health and Longevity.

Curcumin, the active ingredient in the spice turmeric, in particular has real benefit in prostate cancer prevention and treatment.

Another antioxidant of note is grapeseed extract. A 2011 study discovered that grapeseed extract could reduce men's risk of prostate cancer by 40–60%. The extract also has a positive impact on heart diseases. There have not been confirming studies yet.

The realization is that all fresh foods contain lots of antioxidants and, if you are eating well, you are getting plenty of them, especially if you include some of the above-mentioned superfoods in your regular diet. That being said, some of you might want to add antioxidants to your daily regime.

I would suggest foods as your primary source, superfoods next, followed by food-based antioxidant supplements. My best advice is—again and again —to personally test before consuming them. I have found that most recommended antioxidants have a NO test result for me or—at best—test YES for a very short time, which saves me a lot of money. I must be getting what I need from my good diet—and so can you!

Cravings

I've told you about the conditions that create prostate disease, what you need to stop doing and what you need to start doing. One obstacle that often lies in the path of making these types of major lifestyle changes are cravings.

Cravings have many causes. A deficiency in a vital nutrient will easily urge you to crave certain foods. Unfortunately we end up binging on foods that only add to the problem. If you are missing enough good quality sea salt or saturated fats, for example, you could end up eating more and more devitalized breads, cookies and cakes—all of which will add weight and make you less healthy.

Although difficult to digest unless the grain is soaked first, gluten actually leads to cravings. This is because grain products like bread and muffins often contain gluten and produce pleasant feelings and the desire for more. If you have candida and parasites in your gut, then those lead to sugar and starch cravings because sugar and starch are food for those overgrowths.

A lack of saturated fats easily leads to cravings. If you have enough high quality saturated fats, you'll have fewer cravings. We feel satisfied when we eat them, and the cravings stop. The poor quality vegetable fats found in processed and fast foods become addictive because our bodies are never truly satisfied by them. Our bodies crave real food, not food-like substances!

The more you eat sugary foods, the more you will crave. Today many of our manufactured foods also have food additives designed to increase cravings for that product, which cause us to become addicted little by little.

Counting calories makes no sense since so many low caloric foods (i.e., non-foods like artificial sugars) actually are some of the worst offenders. Eating the wrong kind of calories—cakes, cookies or drinks with artificial sugars—simply cause weight gain and a host of problems.

What's the solution to constant cravings and weight gain? Slowly, little by little, start reducing the foods on the STOP list. Eat nourishing real foods instead. You will stop overeating because you will finally get what your body really needs and craves.

Healthy foods will do the trick! Your cravings will disappear as will pounds and pounds of unwanted fat. The *Prostate Cancer Prevention Diet* has real side benefits: a much healthier you!

Conclusion

Remember, superfoods are highly nutritious foods and some of them should definitely be incorporated into your healthy diet. As you are introduced to new foods, personally test whether they would benefit your body or have a negative effect. Just because they're "super" doesn't mean they are super for you!

Some people choose to incorporate superfoods into their diet and skip supplementing all together. In Chapter 9, I discuss the pros and cons of supplementing.

Chapter 9: Supplements for Prostate Health

By far the most important supplement is your daily food! I can't emphasize this enough. Making the right food choices is *the key to health*. Don't let yourself be fooled into thinking that you can make up for poor food choices with supplements.

The complexities and bioavailability of nutrients, enzymes, naturally occurring minerals in food, vitamins, trace minerals (as found in high quality sea salts) and antioxidants found in whole foods cannot be replicated in a laboratory making synthetic versions of these essential ingredients for life. Even natural supplements are a far second to the benefits of natural whole foods eaten daily.

In the short term, if you are unable to take proper care by eating well, then supplements may have a place. But in the long term, your personallytested optimum diet is the secret to your health and the health of your prostate!

Over the years of my search, I took all kinds of supplements, all highly recommended for prostate health. I spent a fortune. Overall with tests, books and supplements, my monthly average was easily $1000 to $2000 (for 10 years!). Most to no avail. That does not mean that supplements will not be effective for you, but they are not the panacea they are often made out to be by slick marketing appeals.

Many well meaning doctors of alternative medicine and their websites as well as some very high quality manufacturers of superb products highly recommend their supplements for optimum health. Their logic, science and research present compelling arguments as to why you need these supplements for your health.

Be wary of these suggestions. Many of these highest quality products will not be beneficial to you and could actually harm you. It does not matter how "good" the product is. The only relevant question is this. Does your body really need them? You will know how to answer this question when you read the chapter on Personal Testing after this one.

I have been unable to tolerate many recommended supplement products at different points in time. Many supplements even caused a severe reaction including complete prostate blockage (see Over-Supplementing in this chapter), and I had to stop them. The theory is that more is better. But sometimes too many herbs or ingredients can cause an irritation. Furthermore, binders and fillers to make them into capsules or tabs can often cause reactions.

Personally test products to see which ones are best for you. It is better to test individual herbs if possible. Look for simpler prostate formulations. Many of the products that I reacted to had great research and the highest quality ingredients (organic or wild). I had to stop taking them.

When you do choose to supplement your diet, here are my rules of the game:

> Use bioavailable natural supplements made from whole foods and herbs.

> Use freeze-dried forms, tinctures, extracts, concentrated or low temperature dried forms, which are closest to the whole foods that we eat.

> Use supplements on a temporary basis, not in the long term, unless it is a concentrated food like cod liver oil.

> Choose organic ingredients whenever possible.

> Avoid synthetic versions found in most commercial grades sold by large mainstream retailers (pharmacies and supermarkets). The quality and digestibility of these are questionable at best and may contain toxins.

> Supplements have become a mega-billion-dollar industry. You can find a huge variety that claim benefits for your prostate and overall health. Supplements can have a varying

> amount of active ingredients,

> quality of ingredients,

> organic or commercial sources,

> natural or synthetic ingredients,

> type of binders or fillers, and/or

> price.

Then, only use a supplement if it tests positive for you.

What to Choose

In order of importance, these are the supplements worth considering when adding supplements to your healthy diet.

Vitamin D

Vitamin D studies show how deficient most people are today in this essential vitamin. **By increasing the amount of vitamin D in your body, you reduce your cancer risk by 50% or more, including prostate cancer!** Vitamin D has many other health benefits. It is the single most important nutrient for your good health. If you are low in it, you are much more prone to a whole range of health conditions.

I urge you to become better informed about sun exposure and vitamin D because they are both so important for your good health (see *Sunlight Exposure* in Chapter 3).

Here are the conservative views of the <u>National Institutes of Health</u>. You will learn more about vitamin D from them but, according to many new studies, their minimum doses are outdated:

> *The results of two studies published in the British Journal of Cancer and Journal of Clinical Oncology found people with higher levels of vitamin D—at the time they were diagnosed—were more likely to survive.*
>
> *Vitamin D New Cancer Hope* by University of Leeds,
> <u>www.leeds.ac.uk/news/article/136/vitamin_d_new_cancer_hope</u>

The articles above reinforce the benefits of moderate sun exposure and adequate vitamin D supplementation when not enough sun is available.

If sun exposure cannot happen because of winter cold, due to dark, cloudy days, or because you lack the time, then the best way to supplement is with food sources like sardines or potent cod liver oil (see next section).

Liposomal Vitamin D3 is another great super high quality alternative. It comes in a liquid and uses a high potency Liposomal delivery that contains true fat for better absorption. This is an excellent way to take your D. For more information, go to the GI for Life website.

The next best choice for vitamin D is natural vitamin D3 supplements, but this is nowhere near as good as the cod liver oil or the liposomal form.

When buying any vitamin D, make sure that you're getting Vitamin D3 (cholecalciferol), not D2, an inactive form of Vitamin D. D2 is about 10 times less effective because it is difficult for the body to absorb and use. Vitamin D3 is fat-soluble, so it is best to take it with some fat or oily food. That's why cod liver oil is so effective!

I prefer 1000 IU capsules of cod liver oil because you can easily personally test how many to take and adjust easily the amount. I took natural D3 before I learned about the benefits of cod liver oil.

Cod Liver Oil

This amazing concentrated food source provides digestible fat-soluble vitamin D plus vitamin A as well as rich amounts of EPA and DHA.

> *Cod liver oil is also rich in eicosapentaenoic acid (EPA) and docasahexaenoic acid (DHA). The body makes these fatty acids from omega-3 linolenic acid. EPA is as an important link in the chain of fatty acids that ultimately results in prostaglandins, localized tissue hormones while DHA is very important for the proper function of the brain and nervous system.*

> *Cod Liver Oil Basics and Recommendations* by S. Fallon and M. Enig, www.westonaprice.org/cod-liver-oil/cod-liver-oil-basics-andrecommendations

Natural cod liver oil is one of the best supplements I have ever taken. I use it in the winter as I live about 300 miles north of Seattle where skies are often grey and overcast for 6 months or more of the year. I use Green Pastures Blue

Ice Royal Capsules, which contain natural cod liver oil, fermented to increase its absorbability, and high-vitamin butter oil. Read more about the combination of fish and butter oils.

It is crucial that you personally test for the optimum quantity you need, and retest regularly to see if the quantity changes, especially as the seasons come and go. I needed 8 capsules per day when I started out (daily recommended dose is 2) and then it reduced over a few weeks to 1–2 per day, and then to none.

Be aware that many varieties of cod liver oil are bleached, which destroys the benefits. Find a high quality one such as those I have recommended above, and ensure you personally test it.

Over-Supplementing

I followed the advice of many natural health practitioners and, as a result, I took a ton of natural supplements every day, sometimes as many as 30–35 different ones per day! In the end, I realized that I was getting worse, and it was costing an arm and a leg to boot! Now that I know how to personally test (see Chapter 10), I have dropped down to 1–2 supplements at most per day, sometimes none. All the other supplements keep giving me a NO test response, although they are the highest quality organic supplements that I could find, including all kinds of antioxidants, that have wonderfully convincing research.

In *Timeless Secrets of Health and Rejuvenation*, Andreas Moritz says that we do **not** need extra vitamins and that they could actually be harmful to our health:

> *Taking extra vitamins can be harmful if the body is unable to make use of them and is left with the additional burden of having to break them down and eliminate them . . . can lead to vitamin poisoning (vitaminosis) which damages the kidneys . . . it would be more healthful and efficient to cleanse the body from accumulated toxins, stored proteins in the blood vessel walls, and impeding gallstones from the liver.*
>
> *To avoid imbalance in one way or the other, you should obtain your antioxidants only from one source—food . . . ideally of organic origin,*

still contain[s] more than enough vitamins to supply the body many times over . . .

The common practice of producing food synthetically and making it 'healthier' by adding synthetically derived vitamins and minerals is at the root of many health problems afflicting both children and adults in the developed world.

Synthetically derived "nutrients" are foreign matter to both animals and humans alike.

Timeless Secrets of Health and Rejuvenation by A. Moritz

I am not saying you should avoid supplements. You just need to personally test to ensure these supplements are useful for you right now, to avoid the possible weakening effects of some supplements and to save money on supplements and invest your money in the best foods you can afford.

I share these views after being a supplement junkie who took recommended vitamins and minerals for years with no positive outcomes. I gave it my best shot for years, yet my prostate just kept getting worse!

I have had reactions to the very best supplements. I never suspected that such abundantly "good" ingredients could cause something as severe as a prostate attack!

If you are relatively healthy, you probably won't have negative reactions like I did. Yet, these products may still be a waste of your money unless you test them to see if they will benefit you.

Now I personally test everything and no longer suffer the difficult side effects that I did before I instituted this practice. In many cases, a supplement will only test YES for a short period, after which it becomes harmful to you. Ideally check out (i.e., personally test) supplements at your health food store before you actually buy them.

Natural vs. Synthetic Vitamins and Minerals

The more I learn about vitamins and minerals, the more convinced I am that it is a mistake to take them in pill form. As I've already said, the best way to get plenty of vitamins is through good eating habits, using sea salt and supplementing with high quality cod liver oil. You will get more than enough vitamins that way.

Your prostate relies on a lot of high quality zinc, magnesium and selenium to stay healthy, and you ain't gettin' it in your Standard American Diet (SAD) of denatured foods!

A healthy prostate contains a higher level of zinc than any other organ in the body. Zinc seems to protect the prostate from prostate diseases by keeping hormone levels in balance. As a bonus, zinc also boosts the immune system by destroying free radicals and bacteria.

This does not mean that you should over-supplement with zinc, which needs to be balanced with some copper. The best way to get zinc is by eating foods rich in zinc like oysters (best), wild salmon, liver (also contains copper), wheat germ, Brazil nuts, egg yolks, sesame and pumpkin seeds, lamb, sea salt (not commercial salt), dark grades of maple syrup and very dark chocolate. Make sure the meat and eggs are from grass-fed animals, not factory-imprisoned, grain-fed animals.

> *There is a large difference between the vitamins found in foods and many of the vitamins sold in pill form in our health food stores and drugstores. Vitamins in foods come with many cofactors—such as related vitamins, enzymes, and minerals—which act with the vitamin to ensure that it is absorbed and properly used . . .*
>
> *Most commercially produced supplements contain vitamins that are either crystalline or synthetic. Crystalline vitamins are those that have been separated from natural sources by chemical means; synthetic vitamins are produced "from scratch" in the laboratory. Both are purified or fractionated concentrates of the vitamin, which act more like drugs than nutrients in the body. They can actually disrupt the body chemistry and cause many imbalances.*
>
> *Nourishing Traditions: The Cookbook that Challenges Politically Correct Nutrition and the Diet Dictocrats* by S. Fallon and M. Enig

In fact, many vitamin and mineral supplements contain artificial additives, synthetic flow agents and chemical colorings that can easily cause reactions in your body.

Eat whole foods and cleanse your body, and you will absorb what you need from your food. Personally test any vitamins and minerals you want to take. Get sun. Add cod liver oil, which is a food, to your diet.

Use the following sources of information to find foods rich in the vitamins and minerals you want (caveat, a few of the foods are not in my "good" list, like soy): Food Sources for Vitamins and Minerals and What Foods Have What Vitamins?

Also, whenever you consider taking a vitamin or mineral supplement, make sure it is made from natural ingredients. Those "experts" who profess that natural or synthetic ingredients are all the same need to read this article: Synthetic vs. Natural Vitamins.

The supplements may be chemically the same, but the effects on the body of the synthetic supplements can be quite different and in some cases very dangerous. The same risks occur in modern foods that add synthetic vitamins or minerals to raise the nutritional profiles. Be very wary of these non-foods. Over time they have a definite health destroying reaction.

Endogenous and Exogenous Supplements

Supplements that are found in common foods or naturally in our bodies are called "endogenous" supplements. Those that are **not** found in our bodies or in common foods are called "exogenous" supplements.

Basically, every food and their derivatives are endogenous, while many herbs are exogenous meaning they lose their benefits after 1–6 months, and you may have reactions to them (if not sooner!).

So when you come across a supplement or herb that you believe may be useful to you, personally test it and retest often. That is the only way to know if a suggestion is going to be good for you. If you get a YES response and the supplement is exogenous, know that you must stop using it at some point. I guarantee you that you will receive a NO test response at some point, and when you do just stop using it.

Some Possible Daily Supplements

Many manufacturers use a multitude of herbs for health supplements or as general antioxidants. These are the main ones:

Supplement	Benefits
Beta Glucan	Antioxidant
Quercitin	Antioxidant
N-Acetyl-Cysteine	Antioxidant
CoQ10	Antioxidant
Lipoic Acid	Antioxidant
Food Enzymes and Probiotics	Digestive aid
FOS	Digestive aid
Acidophilus	Digestive aid
L-Glutamine	Digestive aid
Aloe Vera Juice	Digestive aid
Glucosamine	For bones and joints
PS (Phosphatidyl Serine)	Brain/memory supplement
Acetyl-L-Carnitine	Health enhancer
Lecithin	Protects against many diseases

Specific Prostate Supplements

There are many interesting herbal prostate products on the market today. Most prostate supplements come in capsule form and some as tinctures or teas. You will find many of the ingredients listed below as well as many added vitamins and minerals and some superfood greens.

I find that simpler versions of these supplements give me a YES response when I test, while the concoctions give me a NO. You will have to test to decide.

Prostate Supplement	Benefits
Beta-Sitosterol/Phytosterols	The active ingredient in Saw Palmetto.
Saw Palmetto	The best known prostate herb; many

	studies show that it's a preventative and helps to reduce prostate symptoms.
Pygeum Another well-known prostate herb; many	studies show its benefits for an enlarged prostate.
Nettle leaves	Very popular in Europe to treat BPH; often combined with saw palmetto to relieve BPH symptoms: urgency to urinate, incomplete emptying and constant urge to urinate.
Pumpkin seed extract	Contains high levels of phytates, so be careful
Lycopene	Conflicting research on this one . . . some say it is a useless ingredient as no studies have been done to prove its claims
Soy Isoflavones	Mixed reviews on this one as with soy in general with some saying it is essential for prostate health and others not
Zinc	A crucial prostate mineral: best to eat oysters and other zinc foods (brazil nuts, wild salmon, liver, egg yolks, sea salt, dark maple syrup)
DIM (a phytochemical produced while digesting cruciferous vegetables)	Lowers excess estrogens (eat cruciferous veggies like broccoli)
Pollens	Like rye pollen and others
Small Willow Herb (epilobium parviflorum)	Common prostate herb in Europe

Selenium	An important prostate mineral deficient in our soils and protects against mercury in air and foods. Take 2 soaked, then dried, Brazil nuts daily.

If you are relatively healthy and have only minor symptoms, you may not have any negative reactions to a broad-spectrum prostate supplement. It may work well for you. If you have a more serious condition, then a simpler version or single herb may be the way to go.

Mother Nature Prostate Formulas

Prostate Supplements at Amazon

Saw Palmetto is the most common prostate herb. Some men get relief from using it. Trust your personal test results no matter how incredible the fancy marketing brochures appear! Some claim the whole herb is the best way to go, while others suggest you take the active ingredient in it, as that is more potent.

There can be a world of difference between a whole herb, such as Saw Palmetto, and an isolated and concentrated nutrient taken from it, such as Beta Sitosterol, which often gets promoted as way more potent than the herb itself. I seriously question that assertion because it could be the interaction of different nutrients in the whole herb that is most powerful. Look at this recent article:

The synergy in which phytochemicals affect the human body is complex. Synthetically produced phytochemicals, or nutrients used as pharmaceuticals, do not have the same action as those naturally occurring in the whole food. Plant foods contain a synergy of nutrients and phytochemicals that have potent anti-cancer actions, along with antioxidant and other health promoting effects on the body. The importance of these foods in the diet is undisputed; however, the reductionist medical view of turning nature's perfect food into pharmaceutical drugs misses the point. When isolating compounds unforeseen actions can occur and side effects begin to emerge where they are not seen when consuming the whole plant.

Researchers Believe Plant Based Food Could be Used as an Effective Treatment for Cancer by T. M. Hartle,

www.naturalnews.com/031840_plants_cancer_treatments.html

Dr. Andrew Weil wrote an insightful article on the differences between whole plants and the drugs that are isolated from them:

Using whole-plant remedies is a fundamentally different—and, I would argue, often better—way to treat illness . . . Human beings and plants have co-evolved for millions of years, so it makes perfect sense that our complex bodies would be adapted to absorb needed, beneficial compounds from complex plants and ignore the rest. This is an established fact in nutrition, but the West's sharp distinction between food and medicine somehow blinds us to these properties when it comes to botanicals . . . Plants are (usually) better than pharmaceutical drugs.

Why Plants Are (Usually) Better than Drugs by Dr. A. Weil,
www.huffingtonpost.com/andrew-weil-md/why-plants-are-usuallybe_b_785139.html

For a good tincture of just 3 ingredients, try Prostate Doctor—Native Remedies. I like tinctures for their direct absorption. I also really like this very high quality tincture, Men's Formula, by Baseline Nutritionals.

Another good quality Ayurvedic prostate supplement is Prostate Protection—A Holistic Approach to Prostate Health.

The only way you will know for sure is by personally testing each supplement. (I know I say this a lot, but if you want to save time and lots of money, then personal testing cannot be beat!)

Here is a fascinating supplement, Prostex.

Amino acids are the building blocks of protein, and occur naturally in the body. Prostatic fluid has been found to contain particularly high concentrations of the amino acids glycine, alanine, and glutamic acid, and a special formula of these three substances has been used for decades to treat the urinary symptoms of BPH . . .

While the exact method of action is not fully understood, it is thought that, like other nutritional and herbal supplements, the formula works through a diuretic and anti-edemic effect, reducing excess swelling of prostate and surrounding tissues and encouraging normal urine flow."

Amino Acid Therapy by Prostex, *prostex.com/prostate-guide/aminoacid-therapy/*

Order on their site or here at Amazon, which is a bit cheaper: Advanced Prostex.

Here is a great high density potent supplement you can try: Prost-P10x. This one stands out. Why? Because of the quality and amount of ingredients. They come in an individual day pack inside the bottle. You will find cheaper but none better.

Check out this high potency phytosterol/beta-sitosterol product: NeoProstate.

My bottom line on prostate supps is that they may be helpful for a period, but my experience is that they provide diminishing returns while the highest quality foods seem to supply augmenting returns. Be careful and test!

Here is a source for French Green Clay Capsules that is an inexpensive supplement that also acts as a cleanser to remove toxins from the body:

While many people recognize the benefits of natural clays for skincare, most Americans have yet to experience the age-old European practice of including specialized French Green Clay in the diet. This special form of clay (also known as illite clay) features minerals, trace elements and phytonutrients (which give it its green color). It also absorbs unwanted substances in the GI tract, making it an excellent addition to any detoxification program.

Swanson Premium French Green Clay Natural Detoxifier by Swanson Health Products

Use the following anti-inflammatory herbs in your cooking if they test YES: rosemary, cinnamon, oregano, turmeric, ginger and garlic.

Eat zinc-rich foods like oysters and properly prepared nuts and seeds. Many men are very deficient in zinc, as much as 30-50% of men; the deficiency is worse the older you are. This is a prime driver of prostate problems.

Eat wild not farmed salmon regularly for its omega-3 fatty acids.

Eat cruciferous vegetables (a natural source of DIM used in some supplements) like broccoli, cabbage, Brussels sprouts, kale, bok choy, su choy, collard greens and broccoli sprouts.

> *Sulforaphane from broccoli and cruciferous vegetables selectively destroys cancer cells.*

> *Research details published in the Molecular Nutrition & Food Research journal explains the potent mechanism exhibited by . . . broccoli and cauliflower to ameliorate developing cancer cells. The active photochemical known as sulforaphane targets prostate and other hormone dependent cancer lines and leaves normal healthy cells unaffected.*

> *Sulforaphane from Broccoli and Cruciferous Vegetables Selectively Destroys Cancer Cells* by J. Phillip, www.naturalnews.com/032988_sulforaphane_cancer_cells.html

Other Herbs for the Prostate

Herbs can detox and cleanse the prostate gland, and they can reduce swelling and inflammation by dissolving toxins within the gland. Try some of these:

Peppermint

Peppermint—not spearmint—acts as an anti-inflammatory to the prostate. It may be a useful tea.

Turmeric

This curry spice and herb is an anti-inflammatory and is recommended for prostate cancer treatments. It is available in capsules.

Here are some other prostate herbs:

> Cleavers herb

> Thuja leaf

> Juniper berries

> Corn silk

> Willow herbs (Epilobium parviflorum)—very commonly prescribed in Europe

> Great hairy willow herb (E. hirsutum)

> Uva ursi leaves

> Horsetail (Equisetum arvense)

> Sweet and spotted Joe-Pye rhizome (Eupatorium purpureum and E. maculatum)

> Rye pollen

> Queen Ann's lace (Daucus carota)

> Yellow and white sweet clover herb (Melilotus officinalis and M. alba)

Herbal Prostate Tea

Bell Prostate Ezee Flow Tea is an herbal prostate tea that many men swear by.

Chinese Herbs and Products

You will find many Chinese herbs for the prostate if you search for them. I would look for a product that contains some of the herbs listed on the website below but with my usual caveats—personally test everything (see Chapter 10).

Prostate Health—How to Treat and Prevent Enlarged Prostate with Chinese Herbs

Here are some other Chinese herbal products:

Chinese Prostate Supplement

There is a long tradition of herbal healing in China passed down over the generations. If you live near a Chinatown, then I recommend that you see a Chinese herbal doctor. Just go into various herbal stores and ask them for a Chinese herbal doctor. They will direct you. I have done this on several occasions.

The Chinese herbal doctor will take your pulses to learn your condition and examine your tongue and more as well as ask you questions about your health and diet. From that examination, the Chinese herbal doctor will customize an herbal product for you. It will be weighed and mixed with a variety of herbs with instructions on how to simmer them to make a tonic to drink over the next week or two. Depending on your condition, this can be a very effective treatment for your prostate.

If you do not live near a Chinatown, then you could get an email consultation at Dr. Shen's Chinese Herbs and Medicine (scroll to the bottom of the page at the link).

Herbs work differently from strong medications, which often have dangerous side effects. Herbs work slowly, cleansing and rebuilding, and are more subtle in their effects, but they do have a powerful impact over time. Just because they are herbs does not mean they are good for you! Many will not be so the only thing to do is TEST.

Medical Cannabis

Last, but not least, is medical cannabis (sometimes known as hemp oil, but don't get it confused with the hemp food oil you can find in health food stores!). Medical cannabis is only to be used if you have prostate cancer and to be used in combination with all the dietary changes you need for your optimum nutrition.

This is a potent anti-cancer curing supplement that is starting to be recognized for its medicinal uses, becoming legal in some areas at long last, and finally being made available in the best form to take: as an oil extracted from the potent parts of the plant.

The oil is very thick and gooey like molasses and very powerful. You take it by eating it. A very tiny amount each day.

Watch this excellent documentary of testimonials of real people and the dramatic health improvements they have had.

Conclusion

My advice is rather than supplement, purchase the best quality foods that you can. If you do choose to supplement your diet, use bioavailable natural supplements made from whole foods and herbs, definitely avoid synthetic versions and personally test before consuming. Even better, save yourself a lot of money and test before making the purchase!

In Chapter 10, I finally share my knowledge and experience about personal testing.

Chapter 10: Personal Testing

This chapter is essential if you have a condition and is optional if you are confident that you have found your diet based on the information I have provided already.

The material presented in this chapter is a way to know—with certainty—about any food or supplement you think you want to take, but you want to know if it is beneficial for you or not right now.

Wouldn't it be wonderful to have a reliable way to **know** whether something is healthy for you to eat or use? And to just **know** that you know! In fact, there are simple techniques you can learn that can give you those answers.

Caveat: the techniques to which I'm referring will be very challenging for many readers to accept, especially those of you with a very scientific mindset. I know that personal testing could be easily dismissed as unscientific and not valid.

That would be a mistake.

Why? Because I know it works.

I have had countless examples of being able to discover a problematic food or supplement, which within hours of taking it, caused me very severe reactions including complete inability to urinate. It would have been far better to have tested that item before ingesting it and thus avoiding the problem.

I am a slow learner sometimes, and I have paid the price for that weakness. But I have always been able to find the culprit afterwards by testing all that I ate in my last meal. And many times I have stopped myself from taking something that personally tested NO and thus was able to avoid those reactions.

Suspend your judgment for a moment if you want results! Personal testing works if done correctly. If you have a prostate condition, then testing your inputs is a crucial step to stop the triggers that are worsening your condition.

I call it "personal testing" because you are testing whether something is beneficial for you or not. It has other names as well: muscle testing, behavioral kinesiology, body tuning, energy testing, energy awareness, bioenergetic testing, bio-resonance, pendulum testing, personal dowsing and more. If you have heard these terms before and have negative thoughts about them, please suspend your judgment and read on.

I know very well that many scientists consider dowsing as they do astrology, as a type of ancient superstition. According to my conviction, this is, however, unjustified. . . . Dowsing . . . shows the reaction of the human nervous system to certain factors that are unknown to us at this time. (Albert Einstein) Personal testing can quickly let you know:

> whether a food is good for you or not,

> whether a supplement is conducive to your health or not,

> whether a medication or herbal remedy is good for you or not,

> whether a body care product is good for you or not,

> whether a household product is conducive to your health, or not, and

> how much of an item is optimum to take.

Here's an example: I love chocolate! I have not been able to test positive for months and months. I go into the health food store and test their organic chocolates, and I always get a NO, no matter how much I wish for a YES! I gave up testing chocolate for about a month and, lo and behold, I am now getting a YES for a small amount of 85% dark organic chocolate.

There are no theories or facts about what you should or shouldn't eat. All you need to do is be patient with yourself as you attempt to learn to personally test foods and products. It takes a bit of time, but with persistence, you will develop a skill that is invaluable to have for your health. You will then know what is good for you or not.

What is Personal Testing?

Personal testing involves tapping into your personal awareness or bioenergy by learning to center into your subconscious, which then gives you the answer you are seeking.

We all have that internal guidance system. It comes with being human. In an article entitled "The Intelligence of Your Cells," Dr. Bruce Lipton stated that the conscious mind is capable of processing 40 nerve impulses per second. The subconscious mind can process 40,000,000 nerve impulses per second! Hence, when you personally test, you tap into your inner knowing—subconscious mind—and bring it to conscious awareness.

We all have the ability. The problem is that many of us have lost the ability to tap directly into our inner knowing. Modern life disconnects us from our roots with nature and puts stresses of all kinds on us. The list of reasons that we are disconnected goes on and on.

How many times in your life have you said to yourself, "I'm full, I shouldn't eat any more," and then found yourself dishing up yet another plateful of food? You didn't listen to your body and ate more anyway. The discomfort from being overfull and overfed is ignored.

In the West, we have trained ourselves to stop listening to our bodies' signals and needs. We ignore the feedback mechanisms that are meant to keep us healthy and in balance.

Personal testing gives you a way to tap into that inner wisdom and to learn to listen to what is right for you in this moment. This will help you choose foods and products that are truly health enhancing to help prevent health problems, to speed you on the path to recovery and to heal your prostate if you have a condition.

Some readers may scoff at the techniques for personal testing, possibly because they think it is not scientific. What I can tell you is this: It has worked for me and for thousands of others—there is no cost or drawback to giving this a try.

With an open mind, try the techniques outlined in this chapter. Try it in the quiet comfort of your home, with no one watching, and see what happens. If these techniques work for you, then you have gained an unparalleled tool that will facilitate your health and save you time and money. There is nothing to lose and everything to gain.

All I can say to you, dear reader, is that this skill has saved me from countless agonizing experiences and has speeded me to recovery from a very unhappy prostate. If you are able to put aside your doubts and skepticism and give this an honest try, I believe it will be a boon for you. It will take time and effort to get good at it, but it is worth doing, believe me!

Luckily there are three basic ways to do personal testing, one of which will work well for you.

How to Personally Test

Three basic personal testing techniques that you can use are:

1. muscle testing with a partner,

2. personal muscle testing, and

3. pendulum testing.

Eventually, as your awareness develops and your natural instincts and intuition are strengthened, you may simply know whether something is beneficial for you or not without using testing techniques.

Personally, since I am a very visual person, I love seeing the results of a test and find pendulum testing my favorite. Others who may be more attuned to sensations may find personal muscle testing to be their favorite, while others may enjoy and find they get the best response when testing with a partner.

Whichever test you end up attuning to, let yourself practice more and more. Tell your inner skeptic to take a sabbatical while you test drive personal testing—the benefits are so worthwhile!

Personal testing will also save you a lot of money because you won't buy products that may be wonderful for others, but not for you (at least at this time). You will be able to design your own perfect diet, not one based on some expert's advice (including me!).

I offer you these three methods so that you can find one that you like. There are slight variations on each. Just develop the skill with whichever works best for you. Okay, let's begin!

Muscle Testing with a Partner:

Also known as behavioral kinesiology, this test requires two people: you and your partner, who will test you. The environment should be quiet and calm.

1.   Both of you stand. Your left arm should hang down comfortably atyour side. Your dominant arm (for most people it is their right arm) extends outward in a horizontal position with your elbow fully extended. (If you are left-handed, reverse the arms.)

2.   Your partner should stand behind you. Close your eyes and relaxyour mind. Your partner then places her left hand on your left shoulder to keep you stable, and the fingers of her right hand on top of your right arm over your wrist. Some prefer to face each other, but I think it is best to avoid visual contact.

3.   Your partner will say, "Resist," and then press down quickly on yourarm while you try to resist the pressure. Your partner should do this firmly and smoothly. It is not a contest but rather a way to notice if the arm remains strong or weakens.

4.   Your arm muscle will test strong in this neutral state. If you are in anemotional state or under the influence of drugs or alcohol, it is not a good time to test as you could get mixed results.

5.   Now we want to test something true. Your partner will ask, "Is yourname [insert your name]?" Your arm should remain strong, which is a YES response.

6.   Now your partner will ask a question that will give a negativeresponse, such as, "Is your name Mary?" Your arm will become weak and will descend when pushed down on, which is a NO response.

Now you are ready to test a food or product. Hold the food item in your non-dominant hand (for most people this is the left hand) against your prostate area or solar plexus. Then repeat the arm test. If the product is good for you, your arm will remain strong; if your arm is weak and it collapses, then the product is not good for you at this time. Now you have your answer!

In the case of a supplement that gave you a YES response, you then want to know how much to take. Here is what to do. Start with one capsule in the palm of your hand and test again. If you get a YES, then try 2, then 3. Keep testing until you get a NO. The last YES is your dose for the day. You could take that amount spread over the day (e.g., take one supplement three times if you have three capsules as the daily dose).

In the case of a food like eggs that tested YES, retest with one egg then 2, and so on, to see how many you can eat.

It is wise to retest an item every day to ensure that it is still valid or that the dose doesn't change; this is especially important when you begin using new products. For example, I started testing a new supplement that gave me a YES response. The label advised 2 capsules per day, but I tested for 8! I obviously needed that supplement (cod liver oil)! That dosage lasted for a week. Through repeated testing, I started to reduce the dose per day down to 2 and then 1 capsule. And then for a while, none.

You will have to practice the testing until it becomes easy and natural to you. It is necessary to have an open and calm mind when you do muscle testing. Remember your inner critic is AWL (away with leave)!

This Muscle Testing with a Partner Video is a good video to watch because it demos the basic technique.

Your arm muscles will respond to a particular item either with weakness or with strength, so long as you test properly. Many foods and health products that seem irresistible based on their nutritious contents and marketing will test NO. I find that some wonderful products do this. If you test NO for a product that seems to have many "good" ingredients, it may be because one of the ingredients does not resonate for you. Trust your test results. Move on to something else. Your body may not be able to process or digest it properly, and you do not want to weaken your condition.

Personal Muscle Testing

If you don't have a partner to help you, you can still muscle test alone. There are two ways to do this:

Standing Method

Stand in a relaxed manner and repeat the word "YES" to yourself. Allow your body to move or swing you forward. Now repeat the word "NO," and you will find your whole body moving backwards. Thus, by holding a food or supplement against your prostate area, you will either tilt forward or backward, depending on your body's response to it. Does it resonate or not?

Try the name test: My name is [use your name]. You should swing forward a bit - YES. Then say something false: "My name is [use someone else's name]." The opposite now—NO. You don't need to make the statements aloud—silently is fine. The idea is to train your mind for truth and falsehood, YES and NO. Just practice this for a few minutes a day until it works for you.

Try some seemingly obvious items: see if Coke gives you a YES or NO and then try an orange or carrot. You are ready to test now!

Here is a video for the Standing Personal Muscle Test.

Finger Method

Hold the thumb and first finger of your left hand so they make a circle (reverse if you are left handed). With the index finger of your right hand, you place it inside the circle and say YES, then pull it briskly outward (towards where your thumb and index finger are connected). You should test strong (YES), and you will not be able to open the circle. Now do it with NO and your finger should open the circle.

Do the same name test as above to get your YES and NO responses. Now you are ready to test.

You can then hold the product you want to test against your prostate area or sternum using your arm while you then use your fingers to test. If it is a negative product, your finger will open and exit the circle.

Some testers use different fingers. Use what seems best for you. Here is a video for the Finger Personal Muscle Test.

Pendulum Testing

Pendulum testing is my favorite, and I also believe it can be the most accurate method if used correctly. Pendulum testing requires the use of a pendulum to see your YES and NO responses. What I particularly like is that there is a way to ensure you do not get a false test, like a false positive. That technique will ensure optimum accuracy of your results.

Pendulum testing amplifies your body's awareness and responses to what you are testing.

While a pendulum can be made out of virtually any object that you can hang off of a string, there are better and more responsive pendulums that you can purchase. I believe that getting the best pendulum is well worth the price of around $30—the best purchase of my life!

You will instantly break-even the first time you go to buy a supplement that is supposedly great for you, and you test and get a NO. You will then have recovered the price of the pendulum, and it's free sailing from then on.

To avoid false positives and personal reactions to the device itself, select a pendulum that mimics the shape of the body's energy field, which is egglike. This eliminates many pendulums offered for sale in shops and Internet sites.

The most responsive and accurate device is called the Perfect Pendulum. The people who make and sell Perfect Pendulums are experts in the field of personal energy testing with decades of experience, and I highly recommend these as they are the very best.

Once you master using the pendulum you can then graduate to using your body or hands as the testing device, even more accurately than the above methods. I still have a personal liking for seeing the responses, so I use my pendulum every time I test.

I can easily test with an old nail, nail clippers or exotic drop-shape pendulums with points on the bottom. I have used them all, but none come close to the accuracy and ease of a Perfect Pendulum.

The detailed instructions that come with the Perfect Pendulum are equally as valuable as the pendulum itself. These instructions describe how to use the Perfect Pendulum for different kinds of testing that I have never seen done accurately with the other testing methods. Keep in mind that you cannot ask a question when testing with a pendulum. This technique requires getting a direct YES or NO response to a product or image of it like a photo.

Being made of opaque stone, the Perfect Pendulums are more accurate than glass, wood, plastic or other materials, which helps to avoid switching errors (i.e., when your energy switches back and forth, which will affect your testing responses).

The following information is from the <u>Perfect Pendulum</u> website:

1. *Hold the chain between your thumb and index finger, with the smallball in your palm.*

2. *Deliberately swing the pendulum backwards and forwards with yourwrist dropped rather than straight.*

3. *Have the flat palm of your free hand facing up.*

4. *While watching your pendulum, touch your thumb and index fingertogether—this is called acceptance mudra.*

If your pendulum veers into a circle, this is your YES direction

If it doesn't, open your fingers, wait a few seconds, start the pendulum swinging back and forth again, then close thumb and index finger again while watching your pendulum. Each time you do this, you are clearing your bio-energetic testing circuit

Continue doing this until you get a change of direction with acceptance mudra.

Once you have found your YES direction, you should also practice your NO direction. This is exactly the same process, using acceptance mudra again, but with your palm facing down this time.

Please note: it's very important that you generate your YES and NO directions with the acceptance mudra. Other techniques, such as writing YES and NO on different pieces of paper or asking yourself questions, should not be used.

Testing for switching—the self test: *Before doing any sort of energy testing (with your pendulum, a muscle test etc.), you must first establish whether your energetic 'testing circuits' are flowing properly.*

Your energies can 'switch' often during the day, perhaps as a reaction to a food, a person or being in a certain place. So it is very important to check yourself before using your body as a testing instrument—which is what you are doing when using a pendulum. Many people use pendulums without checking to see if their body is working properly and hence get false or variable results. You can only evaluate the correctness of your answer using a pendulum, if you know that you are reliably getting a 'YES' or a 'NO'.

To do the Self Test, place the Self Test mudra—the thumb pointing out between the two middle fingers of your closed fist—against your heart center. The heart center is approximately two inches up from the bottom of your sternum (breast bone).

A NO means 'not switched', no problems, you can test. A YES means you are switched and must unswitch your circuits before you can use the pendulum or do a muscle test.

<u>Perfect Pendulums Information</u> by The School of Energy Awareness

If you test "switched," just follow the instructions to unswitch. Now that you can get a YES or NO, this is the way I test a product or food. I hold the item against my prostate area and test by swinging the pendulum forwards and back and then it will give me a YES or NO by the direction it then rotates. It's as simple as that.

Below I share with you two videos I made demonstrating personal testing. Before you see these videos, I want to caution you that the motions of your pendulum may be very subtle at the beginning. The turning won't be as strong for you as you see in these videos demonstrating how I personally test foods and products. It may take time for your responses to become as powerful as mine, but even a small movement YES or NO is enough to get your answer.

Part 1: <u>Pendulum Personal Testing—Part 1</u>

Part 2: <u>Pendulum Personal Testing—Part 2</u>

Occasionally, you will get a neutral response, neither a yes nor a no. Nothing happens or what happens is unclear. That means exactly that: the product is neither good nor bad. If you are healthy, then use that product in moderation. If you have a health condition, then I would not use that product unless you feel there is a good reason. When you are stronger, then it will not matter as much. Retest that item later if you want to use it again.

If you find you are having difficulties learning to personally test products then go to <u>Food Energy Awareness Solutions and Training</u> for an online consultation with the experts. These experts can help you learn with specific tips or by testing the foods and supplements that you want. Stephen and Lynda Kane are exceptional in this area. They are the ones who taught me and are the makers of the pendulum that I use.

Another solution is to get the book *Diet Wise* by Dr. Scott-Mumby. You won't need to know how to test but by eliminating many foods, and then adding them back one at a time, you can see which ones trigger a reaction. This will be much harder and more lengthy to do but will work.

Here is another option for you. Take this <u>survey of symptoms</u>. The company will then test 115 foods to find your culprits. But this is far inferior to learning how to personally test.

Personal testing will revolutionize and empower your life.

Try to Set Aside Your Skepticism

I know, it's a bit too wacky for you and over the edge! This writer is too much!

But our subconscious knows what is best for us. Testing just tunes you into a conscious awareness of what you already know.

I know it is surprising, but this approach has consistently worked for me. Many times I've tested an unopened product in a health food store and then retested the same product at home with the actual capsule in my hand, and I got the same YES response.

Personal testing has also worked on something that I sure wished was a YES, but I got a NO response. It was a super sounding prostate supplement, and I wanted to try it, but NO means NO so I passed on it.

On many occasions, I have bought something from the Internet that tested YES from the product image and that still tested the same when it arrived. The last time I did it, I tested the package without opening it after I got it all wrapped from the post office. Then I tested it in the bottle. All times were a YES, including the pill itself.

At times, I have taken a supplement that I didn't or forgot to test because it sounded so good! But later it caused a reaction. My typical reactions are either a sore tongue or frequent urination or worse – none, usually within hours, which indicates a prostate reaction. Then later, I test the supplement and get a NO. If only I had tested sooner!

If you have concerns about a bias or having an agenda, then consider muscle testing with a partner (as shown earlier in this chapter). If you have concerns about people seeing you attempt this in a store, try the Finger Method (also shown earlier in this chapter), as this approach can be very subtle. It looks like you're fidgeting, and no one will even notice you doing it. Frankly, I don't care. I use my pendulum wherever! Most people do not even notice you—they are too concerned with their own shopping.

I know it is hard to put your skepticism aside, but you have nothing to lose and a lot to gain. Try it and see! This has worked like a charm for me and saved me countless dollars and severe reactions, and I hope it works for you too.

Your body's inner wisdom knows what it needs and what you need constantly changes as seasons change, as you change, as your body heals and grows, as certain foods no longer serve you and new foods are needed.

Let's take an example: coffee. Many pundits say it is terrible for you, and others claim that its antioxidants will cure what ails you! So how are you to know? By personally testing, you will get a clear answer for you right now. At the time of this writing, I test YES for organic coffee and NO for the often touted, the-more-you-drink-the-better green tea! In fact, if I drink green tea my body starts reacting to it, and my frequency of urination goes way up while the opposite happens with caffeinated coffee. Go figure!

So who are you to believe? Some guru pundit or your body's own inner wisdom? I know my answer and so will you when you learn how to tune in to your inner subconscious body wisdom.

How do I know personal testing works?

Because I "back-tested" it. I believe my extreme sensitivities to many foods developed because my gut flora had weakened from

> vaccines, which weaken your body;

> antibiotics, which destroy good flora;

> mercury fillings, which leak minute amounts of highly toxic mercury into the body; and

> the anti-nutrient, phytic acid, in many whole natural foods.

I used to wake up in the middle of the night unable to pee—totally blocked! I eventually learned something had triggered the shutdown.

The way that I back-tested was by personal testing everything I had eaten at supper time. I always found something that tested NO—the culprit! And so I started to test foods before I ate them. (That was a simple brain wave!)

I had to give up all that I had learned about diet and the supposedly healthy foods with great profiles and scientific research. The only thing that mattered to me was whether I would react to it—or not.

Real foods like my own garden kale, freshly picked, or apples from my own trees—and many more simple foods—could block me tight so I had to use a catheter to pee! These natural wholesome foods were also culprits at some point: zucchini, beets, organic dairy unless raw, rice and bread, coffee, green tea, all herbal teas and almost all supplements!

Because my symptoms were so observable and so immediate, I became a living laboratory. My health was revolutionized by being able to personally test foods and supplements even of the highest quality and by discovering that many of them would not work for me.

By stopping all the irritants, I was finally able to stop the downslide and begin to heal. Now I can eat many of those former trigger foods—no problem!

Without personal testing, my condition probably would have worsened.

Personal testing is the most important health discovery of all time in my opinion because it allows you to know what works for you—no theories, no guesswork, no must do's. You know. Period.

Personal Testing Theory

If you want to learn how this works, read more here: <u>Energy Medicine</u> or <u>Muscle Testing</u>. And this book, <u>Blinded by Science</u>, explains many mysteries of nature so you can understand how it works as well.

How personal testing works through a closed package or bottle is a mystery to me, but again it does work. I can live with uncertainty about how it works because it has proven, without a shadow of a doubt, to work for me. It removes all the guesswork from my choices about other experts' recommendations. I just personally test each item and get my answer.

Testing Tips

When you get a YES for something new, retest it again regularly to ensure that the product is still good for you, especially if you have many sensitivities or if you are healing.

You can calm your mind and enhance your testing by placing your tongue up to touch the roof of your mouth behind your top teeth (an advanced meditation technique) and then swallow. Then test with whatever method you choose. When you get good at testing, it will only take a few seconds to get a response.

Remember no matter how "good" for you a food or supplement is, whether recommended in this book or elsewhere, if you have too much of it, then it can easily change to "bad" for you! It has happened to me many times —with ghee, miso, sauerkraut, saw palmetto, selenium, greens, flax oil and more!

As you cleanse, detox and start to heal, your sensitivity to foods and supplements goes up. Your body knows what it needs. Set aside your opinions and personally test (and retest). You will then know what is healthy for you to eat or not. As you get healthier and your sensitivity diminishes, you find that you have fewer reactions.

Conclusion

Each one of us is so unique that we need these tools to **know** what is best for us. It is easy to learn one (or more) of these tests, and this skill will empower you to make the right health decisions for you.

Personal testing will revolutionize your health by going beyond the advice and recommendations of others—no matter how qualified or eminent they are. Testing goes beyond the selling points of a product or the ideas someone else has for you about what you "need" or what you "should" eat. Testing allows you to know for sure.

Take all the good advice that comes your way and put it to good use by testing and making decisions based on your true knowing.

Chapter 11: Conclusion

Are all of these changes too much?

Tell me which you would prefer: getting healthy by spending more time and money on your health and well-being **or** getting sicker and being medically treated with the real risks of side effects (downplayed by doctors), such as being unable to get erections or wearing adult diapers?

When you eat only what your body truly wants and needs, then you can prevent prostate cancer from being an issue in your life. Little by little, chronic conditions and food reactions will start to subside so healing can begin.

We live in a world of great complexity and have the benefit in the West of access to a wide range of foods and supplements. The keys to health are to embrace a diet rich in whole natural foods and nutrients, to learn how to prepare foods using time tested traditional methods that enhance digestibility and vitamin mineral absorption, and to supplement wisely with the highest quality natural ingredients that you personally test to reveal a need in your body.

By doing these things, you will avoid the mistake that so many men make of thinking that more is better when they are actually harming themselves because they do not know what is best for them nor what their specific and unique dietary needs are.

Lastly, remember, you must stop those foods that can lead to prostate cancer and replace them with healthy ones that nourish you and your prostate. There are no shortcuts. Just good changes and little by little you will get better and prevent chronic prostate problems.

My hope is that you have learned or gleaned some useful insights. For me it is easy to give up bad habits, uninformed opinions and advice from pundits. When you know the impact on your health, it's easy to start discovering real foods and to give up unhealthy manufactured concoctions.

If you make healthy eating a priority in your life, it will be perhaps the most important decision you can make. Yes, it will cost you as you give up your old bad habits and will demand time, money and energy. But the rewards are infinite: a renewed life, a more direct connection to the joys and abundance of nature and a diet that will ensure not only great prostate health but also sexual and overall vitality for years.

~~~~~~
~~~~~~